# NAVIGATING LUNG CANCER
## 360° OF HOPE

### 3RD EDITION

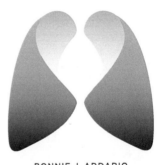

BONNIE J. ADDARIO
**LUNG CANCER**
FOUNDATION

The Bonnie J. Addario Lung Cancer Foundation (ALCF) was founded in 2006, but it really began long before its official start date when Bonnie received a Lung Cancer diagnosis and her life was redefined. Her prognosis was grim when she was diagnosed in 2004. Following a 14-hour surgery, a battery of nurses and doctors, an army of radiation and chemotherapy treatments, blood clots, procedures and tubes that invaded her formerly predictable life, Bonnie became a Lung Cancer survivor.

In a unique position to become the voice for the other 1.5 million people personally affected by the number one cancer killer, she began to think of ways to help people facing the crisis of this highly stigmatized disease. "What about the 450 patients who die each day of Lung Cancer in the U.S. alone and their families?" Bonnie asked. "Where's the outrage?" On March 6, 2006, the news broke that Dana Reeve lost her battle with Lung Cancer. Bonnie decided:

# "Enough was enough!" ALCF was born.

Since it's founding, ALCF has grown into the first international collaborative entity of its kind, raising millions of dollars for Lung Cancer research and programs to support patients and their families.

ALCF has also grown to include ALCMI, an international research consortium, Jill's Legacy, an advisory board of promising young professionals, as well as our family of affiliates, independent fundraisers and partners.

www.lungcancerfoundation.org

# AUTHORS

**Bonnie J. Addario, Founder & Survivor**
Bonnie J. Addario Lung Cancer Foundation

**Shane P. Dormady, MD, PhD Editor-in-Chief**
Valley Medical Oncology Consultants

Associate Executive Director of Patient Services and Programs
Senior Writer / Editor
Project Manager / Contributing Writer

**Danielle Hicks**
**Eileen Johnson, RN, MSN, CPHQ**
**Alicia Sable-Hunt, RN, MBA**

# AUTHORS / ADVISORY BOARD

**Lisa Boohar, MD**
Medical Director at Sequoia Hospital, Department of Radiation Oncology

**Elizabeth A. David, MD**
Assistant Professor of Surgery, Thoracic Surgeon at University of California Davis

**Shane P. Dormady, MD, PhD**
Director of Thoracic Medical Oncology at El Camino Cancer Center
Valley Medical Oncology Consultants

**David R. Gandara, MD**
Professor of Medicine at the University of California, Davis School of Medicine and
Associate Director of Clinical Research, and Director of Thoracic Oncology
UC Davis Comprehensive Cancer Center

**Paul Hesketh, MD**
Director of Thoracic Oncology Sophia Gordon Cancer Center and Director of Thoracic Oncology
Lahey Clinic Medical Center

**Richard Lanman, MD**
Chief Medical Office, Guardant Health

**Robert Sinha, MD**
Medical Director, El Camino Hospital Radiation Oncology

# CONTRIBUTING AUTHORS

**D. Ross Camidge, MD, PhD**
Director, Thoracic Oncology Clinical and Clinical Research Programs and Attending Physician
within the Developmental Therapeutics Program, University of Colorado Cancer Center

**Guneet Walia, PhD**
Senior Director of Research & Medical Affairs, Bonnie J. Addario Lung Cancer Foundation

**For Additional Copies:** To order additional copies go to www.lungcancerfoundation.org, call us at 1-650-598-2857 or email hope@lungcancerfoundation.org.

Bonnie J. Addario Lung Cancer Foundation • 1100 Industrial Road #1 • San Carlos, CA 94070
**Design: White Space, Inc.**

# ACKNOWLEDGMENTS

The Bonnie J. Addario Lung Cancer Foundation (ALCF) is proud to publish the 3rd Edition of *Navigating Lung Cancer 360° of Hope* with the most recent advancements and updates to help patients in real time. We are eternally grateful to Dr. Shane Dormady for his leadership and expertise editing this guidebook and to the leading lung cancer clinicians who provided insight and direction on the original content.

It is only through the generosity of our supporters that we are able to publish and re-publish this guidebook and offer it free of charge to the lung cancer community, lung cancer patients and their families. For this 3rd edition, special thanks goes to Boehringer Ingelheim, Celgene, Genentech, Merck and Novartis. Past edition support included Accuray®, Bodesix, Cancer Commons, Caris Life Sciences®, Covidien-Inreventional Lung Solutions, Genetech and GTx®. Visit "Our Generous Supporters" chapter located at the back for more information on products and services that benefit the lung cancer community.

If you or your company would like information on supporting future editions, please contact Samantha Cummis: sam@lungcancerfoundation.org.

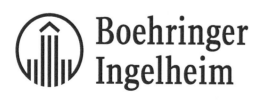

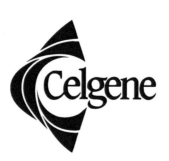

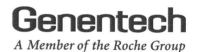

Dear Patients,

I have been with the Bonnie J. Addario Lung Cancer Foundation (ALCF) from its beginning in 2006 and I am honored to help them lead patients to the best possible outcomes.

If you are holding this handbook or reading it online, you've taken the first best step to connecting yourself with the most experienced clinicians worldwide and with a foundation that provides the information you need on your cancer journey.

One of the most important resources that ALCF provides in the Living Room. On the third Tuesday of every month, you can tune into the lungcancerlivingroom.org to meet other patients who are either exactly where you are or years ahead and LIVING with lung cancer—patients all over the world. I have spoken many times over the years at the Living Room, am a co-author of this handbook, and am part of a team of leaders in lung cancer who support this foundation and its patients. ALCF is a lifeline for many of my patients and we are all here to help you and your family in every way we can.

It's important to know that there are many, many kinds of lung cancer. It's complex. The way we approach lung cancer today, as opposed to 10 years ago, is through personalized medicine and individualized care, because each of you is different.

The pace of advancement and learning new things in lung cancer has never been faster than it is today. More and more, lung cancer is a poster child for all the other cancers where we can take the information from the laboratory and translate it into how we take care of patients. All of us need to have our running shoes on if we're going to keep up. Today, when something is found in the laboratory it takes less than a year to make its way to the clinic and right to the patient.

From the start, getting information must be part of your lung cancer journey. Most of my patients are informed before they come to see me. Sometimes they pick up bad information, but by and large they know a lot. Having knowledgeable patients make decisions together with their doctors, as a partnership, is very positive approach for both patients and physicians. It is important for you to know that often, there are options, not always right or wrong answers.

You are a patient who now holds in your hands a resource that is your best first step toward understanding and living with lung cancer. In this book and through the lung cancer Living Room you will become educated, informed and most important…you will find answers, directions, options and HOPE.

What we want all our patients to do is live their lives every day to the fullest.

Warmly,

David R. Gandara, MD
Professor of Medicine at the University of California, Davis School of Medicine and
Associate Director of Clinical Research, and Director of Thoracic Oncology
UC Davis Comprehensive Cancer Center

# 26 Questions to Ask Your Physician:

1. What type of lung cancer do I have?

2. How does the type of cancer I have affect my treatment options?

3. What stage is my cancer?

4. How does that affect my treatment options?

5. Has my biopsy tissue been sent out for genomic/molecular testing?

6. What is the difference between lung specific (EGFR, EML4-ALK, ROS1) and next generation sequencing?

7. Which testing was my tissue sent out for and how is that decided?

8. If the testing is positive, what are my treatment options?

9. If the testing is negative, what are my treatment options?

10. How can I learn more about my treatment options? ie: Chemo, Surgery and Radiation

11. If the best treatment for me is not covered by my insurance, what resources are available to help with access/payment?

12. Are there any Clinical Trials I should consider?

13. What cancer centers or Universities are specializing in my type of cancer?

14. Can I get a second opinion at one of these centers and still be treated here locally by you?

15. How long will I be on treatment before I know it is working?

16. How often are my follow up scans?

17. When should we re-biopsy and is liquid biopsy an option for me?

18. What are the side effects of my treatment?

19. How are these side effects managed?

20. I want children in my future, should I consider fertility preservation before starting treatment?

21. Will my treatment affect my daily routine?

22. Can I still work during treatment?

23. Can I travel during treatment?

24. Will I need oxygen to fly or if I am traveling to high altitudes?

25. What resources are provided for people with lung cancer?

26. Who is my contact person here for any questions I may have?

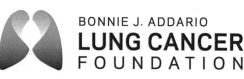

BONNIE J. ADDARIO
**LUNG CANCER**
F O U N D A T I O N

# TO EVERYONE TOUCHED BY LUNG CANCER,

I was diagnosed with lung cancer at the age of 56. I was a wife, a mother, a grandmother, business woman, and one of millions of Americans diagnosed with lung cancer. Faced with a 16% survival rate[1] and following a 14-hour surgery, radiation and chemotherapy treatments that invaded my formerly predictable world, I became a lung cancer survivor with a *new purpose* in life.

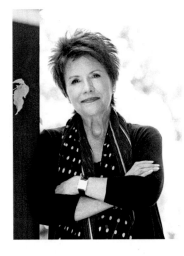

Despite losing three family members to lung cancer, when the doctor said, "you have lung cancer," I realized I knew very little about the disease. So, I searched for information. I was surprised by how difficult it was to find credible information on lung cancer, treatment options, and how to live with cancer. Everyone kept saying that "cancer is a journey" but no one could provide me with a roadmap. I was lost and I was only just diagnosed.

In 2006, the ALCF was founded to empower those diagnosed with lung cancer through education and to fund novel research efforts that directly impact patients, *today*. Our innovative patient education programs are designed and led by lung cancer experts with the goal of supporting you and your family throughout your diagnosis. We support promising research projects through our grants program and the formation of the Addario Lung Cancer Medical Institute (ALCMI). To date, we have raised over $30 million and dedicated approximately 90% to novel research projects, patient education programs and lung cancer awareness.

The **3rd Edition of this guidebook** is the culmination of years of research, conversations with lung cancer experts and patients, and my personal experience. It is designed to be a resource throughout your cancer journey whether you are newly diagnosed, facing a relapse, or a loved one of someone living with lung cancer. You will find questions to pose to your doctor, detailed explanations of complex treatment options, and access to additional resources in the cancer community.

Lung cancer research is advancing rapidly. In the past two years alone, we have seen new drugs brought to market, many clinical trials started across the nation, the advancement of molecular testing, and better side effect management. All of which is needed to improve lung cancer survivability. To this end, we are committed to keeping this guidebook updated with the latest information available.

It is my greatest hope that this guidebook is helpful to you throughout your cancer journey and that we have a positive impact on your life. If I can leave you with one message, it is that you are not alone. Visit our website, join one of our support groups or fundraisers, or simply call us—we are here to help you throughout your journey.

With love,

Bonnie J. Addario, Lung Cancer Survivor
Founder of the Bonnie J. Addario Lung Cancer Foundation
& Addario Lung Cancer Medical Institute (ALCMI)

"The most comprehensive
and accessible resource available for
lung cancer patients."
—Arlene, Survivor

*This guidebook is dedicated to
all lung cancer patients
and their families and friends.*

As vital information becomes available,
new print editions of this guidebook will be released
with updated PDFs available on our website and
through our mobile app.
*Check our website (www.lungcancerfoundation.org) or
Amazon.com to make sure you have
the most current edition.*

# TABLE OF CONTENTS

**LUNGCANCERREGISTRY.ORG**

The Lung Cancer Registry was created for ANYONE who has been diagnosed with lung cancer to help researchers better understand the disease and develop better treatments.

More than 1.8 million people in the world are diagnosed with some form of lung cancer every year. And, though there has been progress in treatment options, it is not enough. As a member of the Lung Cancer Registry, you become a part of a global effort to better understand the disease, and your history is an important tool in developing new therapies.

The registry allows patients to be part of the solution. The data gathering can lead to big research, and that is a big deal.

When researchers study lots and lots of health data from you and thousands of others living with lung cancer, they can see patterns. Those patterns could lead to better understanding, diagnostic techniques and treatments—and ultimately better outcomes.

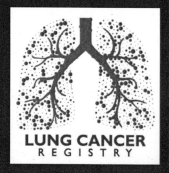

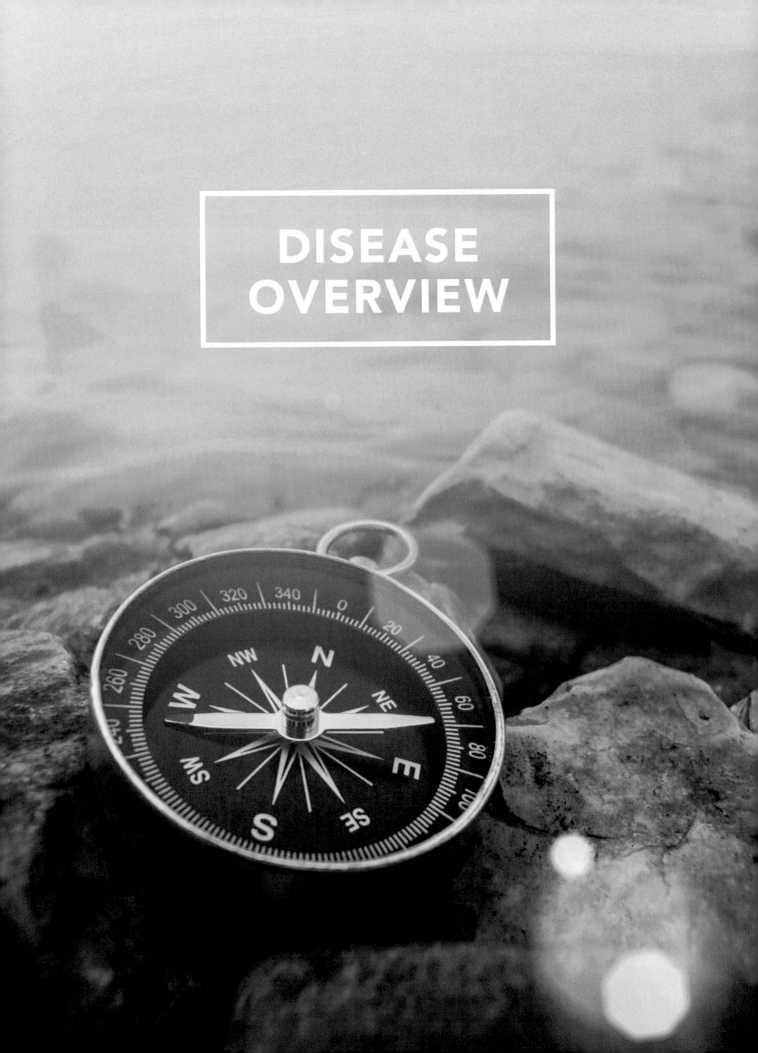

*My cancer center gave me information regarding the Bonnie J. Addario Lung Cancer Foundation and the Patient Education Handbook as soon as I was diagnosed with lung cancer. As the diagnosis process continued to find out type, stage and genomic mutation I would reference the handbook throughout my appointments and procedures.*

*I got hope after meeting several stage IV lung cancer survivors and speaking with Bonnie at the World Conference on Lung Cancer Pancake Walk. The event just so happened to be a drive away in Denver, just weeks after my lung cancer diagnosis. I framed photos from that day. When I look at them it brings back that initial feeling of hope.*

*—Lisa Moran, survivor*

# DISEASE OVERVIEW

After you receive a diagnosis of lung cancer, it is normal to feel scared and alone. We want to help you understand your disease, what you can do to help take care of yourself, and what we can do to help you. This guidebook will help you know what to expect during this process. We know that having information when you need it is critical; however, this guidebook will <u>not</u> replace your interactions with your healthcare team.

### What is lung cancer?

In a healthy body, normal cells grow, mature, and eventually die and are replaced by other healthy cells. Occasionally, abnormal cells in the body begin to develop and grow. If your body recognizes these cells as "abnormal," the body's defense mechanisms may kick into action to destroy the abnormal cells much the same as when bacteria are destroyed by white blood cells. In the case of cancer, your body sees these abnormal cells as part of your body, so it does not attack them and as a result, the cells begin to grow out of control.

*DNA*, which stands for deoxyribonucleic acid, is the molecule in every cell that controls how that cell grows and functions. In a cancer cell, the DNA is damaged and is reproduced in other abnormal cells. In most types of cancer, these abnormal cells begin to stick together and form *tumors*. Tumors are usually classified as *benign* (non-cancerous) or *malignant* (cancerous).

When we talk about lung cancer, we are talking about this out-of-control, malignant growth that starts in the lung tissue. As the cancer cells grow and multiply, the normal cells in the lung are replaced by the malignant cells.

Cancer cells can develop in any part of the body and then spread to other parts of the body through the blood and lymph systems. When this happens, the cancer is said to have metastasized and the resulting tumors are called metastatic *tumors* or metastases. Lung cancer that starts in the lung is called *primary lung cancer*; if the cancer started in another part of the body and metastasizes to the lung, it is called *secondary lung cancer*.

The *lymphatic system* (or lymph system for short) is a system much like the blood system in the body. The lymph system is responsible for carrying nutrients to the cells and waste away from the cells. The *lymph nodes* are special parts of the lymph system that are responsible for filtering the wastes out of the liquid that passes through. When waste collects in the lymph node, it swells and becomes painful. These lymph nodes are in many different places in your body. That is why your doctor and nurses will feel around your neck, in your armpits, in your groin and other areas. They are looking for these swollen glands.

**What causes lung cancer?**
Primary lung cancer is caused by the out-of-control growth of cells that do not die as in the normal cell pattern. The cause of lung cancer may not always be known.

*Carcinogens* are those things that can cause cancer. Normal cells in the lung can be affected by carcinogens in the environment, genetic factors, or a combination of those factors. Exposure to carcinogens may form molecules in the body called *free radicals* which damage cells and alter the DNA of the cell. This damage may cause cancer.

Environmental factors include things such as smoking, secondhand smoke, radon gas, air pollutants, asbestos, heavy metals, and chronic dust exposure. Genetic factors may include an inherited (passed from parent to child) or a genomic mutation. A *genomic*

*mutation* is damage to the gene that increases the chances of developing a particular kind of cancer.

## What are the signs and symptoms of lung cancer?

It is important to recognize the signs and symptoms of lung cancer in order to ensure a reliable diagnosis. A sign is something that can be seen by someone else; for example, a rash is a clinical sign. A symptom is something that cannot be seen by someone else but must be described by the person; for example, a headache is a symptom. Early in the disease, lung cancer may not produce any signs or symptoms. However, as the disease progresses, certain key signs and symptoms may develop. Possible signs and symptoms of lung cancer may include:

- A cough that does not seem to be related to a specific illness, a change in a chronic cough, or a cough that does not go away
- Shortness of breath particularly if it is not related to physical activity or if the shortness of breath seems worse than it should be for the amount of activity ("I walk to the corner and have to sit down and catch my breath before I can walk back")
- New wheezing that is unrelated to a specific illness ("When I breathe, it sounds like I'm whistling")
- Coughing up blood (*hemoptysis*)
- Chest pain
- A hoarse voice or a marked change in voice
- Chronic fatigue ("I just can't seem to get enough rest; I'm always tired")
- Weight loss with no known cause
- Headaches
- Painful lumps in the neck, armpits, or groin caused by inflammation of the lymph glands as the cancer spreads through the lymphatic system

11

All of these signs and symptoms can be caused by other diseases and conditions and may not indicate a diagnosis of lung cancer. However, when several of these symptoms exist, particularly if they do not get better in a short period of time, you should visit your healthcare provider for diagnosis and treatment.

**What should I ask my healthcare provider?**
We understand that this is a scary time for you and your family and we want you to know that we are here to help.

Before your first appointment with your doctor, and at every appointment after that, be prepared with a written list of questions. Between appointments, keep a pad of paper and pencil with you so that you are always ready to jot down a question that comes to mind. At every appointment, ask all of your questions and ask for clarification when the healthcare provider gives an answer you don't understand. Write down the answer to each question. Read the answers back to your provider to make sure you have recorded the information correctly. If possible, take a friend or spouse with you to each appointment. Two sets of ears and two brains are more likely to hear and remember all the information. If your healthcare provider agrees, it might be helpful to take a tape recorder to the appointment and record the discussion.

> Throughout this guidebook, you will find suggested questions or points to discuss with your healthcare team in boxes like this one.

**Are there different types of lung cancer?**
Five types of lung cancer have been identified: Non-small cell lung carcinoma (NSCLC), small cell lung carcinoma (SCLC), mesothelioma, carcinoid, and sarcoma. NSCLC and SCLC represent about 96% of all lung cancers. These two types of lung cancer are identified by the size of abnormal cells and the way the cancer spreads in the body.

Treatments for these two types of cancer are different so it is critical that the type of cancer is correctly identified.

## Non-Small Cell Lung Cancer (NSCLC)

*NSCLC represents about 85 to 90% of all lung cancers[2] and can be further described as:*

- *Adenocarcinoma*
- *Epidermoid or squamous cell carcinoma*
- *Pancoast or pulmonary sulcus tumor*
- *Large cell undifferentiated carcinoma*

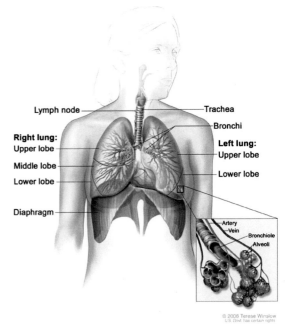

**Adenocarcinoma:** Adenocarcinoma is the most common type of lung cancer accounting for 40% of all cases.[2] Typically, this type of lung cancer starts growing in tissue on the outside surface of the lung. The tumor in a lung adenocarcinoma is made up of cells that tend to line up in small masses. These tumors vary in size and how fast they grow.

Bronchioloalveolar carcinoma, or BAC, is a type of adenocarcinoma that is generally considered to be resistant to, or not killed by, chemotherapy. BAC tumors account for 2 to 6% of all lung cancer and are often found in women who have never smoked.[3]

Often, Asians are affected more often than other ethnic groups. Surgery seems to be the only treatment that may cure BAC tumors. If you have a BAC tumor, the rate of long-term survival might be higher than other NSCLC tumors.

**Epidermoid or Squamous Carcinoma:** Epidermoid or squamous cell carcinoma is the second most common type of lung cancer and is responsible for about 25 to 30% of cases.[2] Usually, this cancer starts growing in one of the large *bronchi* of the lung; the bronchi are the large breathing tubes that connect the *trachea*, or windpipe, to the lungs. The squamous cell carcinomas tend to grow more slowly than other types of lung cancers.

**Pancoast Tumor:** A Pancoast tumor is sometimes called a pulmonary or superior sulcus tumor. Typically, this type of lung cancer is found at the top of the lung and has a tendency to spread to ribs and bones of the spine. Since the Pancoast tumor usually grows on the top of the lung, it is very close to nerves and the spine; these facts make surgery on these tumors very difficult. Pancoast tumors account for fewer than 5% of all primary lung cancers.[2]

**Large Cell Undifferentiated Carcinoma:** Large cell undifferentiated carcinoma is so named because it cannot be identified as one of the other NSCLC types. This form of lung cancer is responsible for about 10 to 15% of all cases and is likely to be found in any part of the lung.[2] The large cell undifferentiated carcinoma is aggressive meaning it tends to grow and spread rapidly.

## Small Cell Lung Cancer (SCLC)

SCLC represents about 10 to 15% of all lung cancers.[2] These lung cancers typically grow rapidly and are aggressive forms of lung cancer. SCLC can be further defined as small cell carcinoma (oat cell cancer) or combined small cell carcinoma. In addition, SCLC is usually described as limited or extensive.

SCLC tumors may also cause *paraneoplastic syndromes*. A paraneoplastic syndrome is a collection of symptoms that develops as a result of cancer but is not directly related to the cancer cells. Usually, these symptoms are caused when the SCLC tumor produces hormones or other specialized proteins that cause an inflammatory response in the body. The body's immune system reacts to these substances and can begin attacking normal nervous system cells causing problems in the nervous system.

## Lung Mesothelioma

Malignant lung mesothelioma is diagnosed in 2,000 to 3,000 people in the United States each year.[4] The *mesothelium* is the lining that covers the body's internal organs and cavities. This rare form of cancer is most commonly found in the *pleura*, or outer lining, of the lungs and internal lining of the chest wall thus the name "lung mesothelioma." Pleural mesothelioma accounts for approximately 70% of all mesothelioma cases.[5] For more information on this disease, visit the National Cancer Institute at http://www.cancer.gov/cancertopics/pdq/treatment/malignantmesothelioma/patient.

## Carcinoid

Carcinoid tumors in the lungs are extremely rare representing about 1% of all lung cancer cases.[6] Carcinoid tumors grow slowly in the lining of the lungs. Because the carcinoid tumors are composed of endocrine cells and secrete hormones, they are often consider endocrine tumors. These very slow growing carcinoid tumors can often be treated with radiation, surgery, chemotherapy and immunotherapy. People with certain genetic disorders (multiple endocrine neoplasia type 1 and neurofibromatosis type 1) may be at a higher risk of developing carcinoid tumors.

## Sarcoma

Sarcoma is another extremely rare cancer that is seen in about 1% of all lung cancers. Typically, a sarcoma is found in bone or other soft tissues. The sarcoma is different from other tumors because of the cells in which it grows. For more information on sarcoma, visit the Sarcoma Foundation of America at http://www.curesarcoma.org/index.php/patient_resources/.[7]

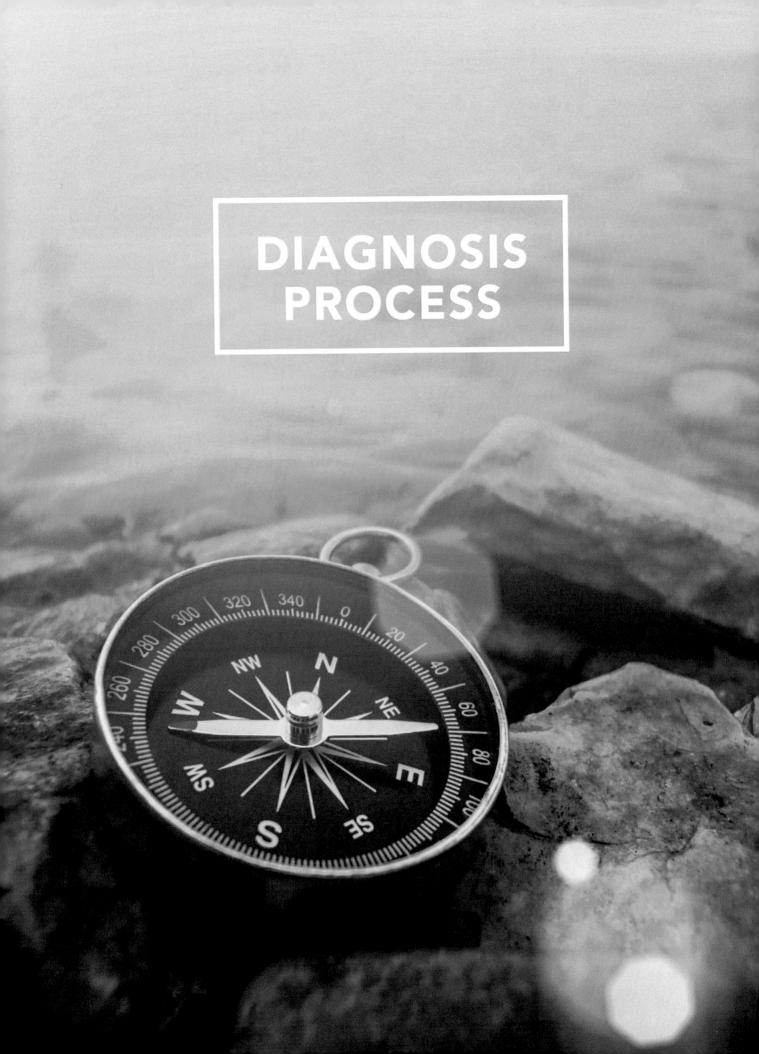

# DIAGNOSIS PROCESS

*This handbook is an invaluable guide to the world of lung cancer. It creates a sense of knowledge and understanding when it comes to the brash new reality you and loved ones are now living. It's a comprehensive guide that gives you the security of knowledge in an overwhelming situation—a great place to begin your path to recovery and wellness. Find easy to comprehend definitions that lay a foundation of understanding to help construct a plan that is best-suited for you in this journey.*

*The foundation is a warm embrace when you feel like you're in free fall. With the compassion of a saint, the tenacity of a bulldog, and the strength of an army, Every single staff member is sincerely here for you and wants the very best for you and your loved ones. I'm so blessed to have the resources of the Lung Cancer Foundation. They are a wonderful support system and definitely someone you want on your team!*

*—Bekah, survivor*

# DIAGNOSIS PROCESS

**My doctor found a spot on my lung –**
**What happens next?**
First, take a deep breath and know that this spot may not be lung cancer; it may be something such as a benign (non-cancerous) nodule, infection, or many other things. The next steps in the process will help your doctor determine, or diagnose, the problem.

Your doctor will talk to you about what tests will be done to determine if the spot is cancer. Usually, your plan will include some sort of radiographic, or x-ray, tests. Your doctor may also want to do a biopsy of the spot. A biopsy involves taking a tissue sample from the area on or around the lung and examining it under a microscope.

> Questions to ask your physician during the diagnosis process:
> - What tests will I need to determine if I have lung cancer?
> - Should I watch and wait?
> - If I decide to watch and wait, how long before you check the spot or nodule again?
> - What is active surveillance?
> - What are the chances the spot or nodule is benign (non-cancerous)?
> - Do I need x-ray tests?
> - Do I need a biopsy?
> - How long will it take to get my biopsy results?
> - What will each test show?

## RADIOGRAPHIC TESTS

The radiographic, or x-ray, tests described here are not painful. The most painful thing you will experience during these tests is a needle stick for those tests that require an injection of a radioactive liquid.

**Computed Tomography (CAT or CT Scan):** A CAT or CT scan is done using a special x-ray machine that gives a more detailed picture inside your body than a normal chest x-ray. CT scans can find very small tumors in the lung and can help to determine if the cancer has spread to the lymph nodes around the lungs. This scan will help your doctor know what size the tumor is and the exact location of the tumor.

**Positron Emission Tomography Scan (PET Scan):** A PET scan is done by another very specialized machine that rotates around your body giving a three dimensional view of your body and allowing your doctors to see the differences between malignant and benign areas. Before the PET scan, a member of your healthcare team will inject a small amount of sugar water with radioactive isotopes into a vein. A radioactive isotope is an atom that emits radiation that can be "seen" by the radiological equipment. As the PET scanner rotates, it shows a picture of where the isotopes are deposited in the cells. Malignant tumors show up brighter in the scan because the cancer cells are more active and are using more of the sugar water mixture than normal cells do.

**Magnetic Resonance Imaging (MRI):** The MRI uses huge magnets, magnetic fields, and radio waves to create clear images of many different areas of the body such as the brain, muscles, joints, and blood vessels. Before this test, the x-ray technician will ask you to remove all metal (rings, glasses, bracelets, etc.) that may be attracted to the magnets.

> If you are diagnosed with stage IV lung cancer, ask your doctor if it is appropriate to receive a brain MRI to check for metastases.

**Bone Scan:** A bone scan is a very specific test that may be used to determine if cancer has spread to the bones. Again, with this test, the radiology technician will inject a small amount of sugar water with a radioactive isotope solution into your vein. This fluid begins to accumulate in areas of abnormal bone growth where a radiation scanner can measure the radioactivity levels and record them on x-ray film providing a clear picture of areas that might have cancerous tumors.

## BIOPSY PROCEDURES

You will want to discuss the biopsy procedures listed here with your physician to understand which procedures are necessary in your unique situation. We have highlighted several points to discuss with your doctor to help you get the information you need to make informed decisions about your care.

**Fine Needle Aspiration (FNA)** is usually performed by an interventional radiologist (a doctor who specializes in doing procedures using radiology) or pulmonologist (a doctor who specializes in lung disease). In this procedure, the doctor will insert a needle through the chest wall into the tumor. Cells from the tumor are pulled into the syringe and are then examined by a pathologist under a microscope. The pathologist is the doctor on your team who specializes in diagnosing disease by examining tissue and body fluids. The fine needle aspiration procedure is done with the help of a CT scanner, fluoroscopy (live x-ray images done using a fluoroscope) or MRI to guide the needle to the exact location of the tumor. Before this procedure, the biopsy site (area that will be stuck by the needle) is numbed so the procedure should not hurt.

> It is important to obtain enough tumor tissue for diagnosis and molecular testing. Ask your doctor if an FNA biopsy will collect enough tissue for both diagnosis and molecular testing.

**Core Needle Biopsy** is usually performed by an interventional radiologist or pulmonologist. This procedure is similar to the FNA, but the doctor can usually get a larger piece of tissue with core needle biopsy. Using this method, the pathologist will have enough tissue to determine the type of lung cancer and for molecular testing. The core needle biopsy is usually done with the aid of some sort of x-ray equipment to guide the needle to the exact location of the tumor. Again, before this procedure, the biopsy site (area that will be stuck by the needle) is numbed so the procedure should cause minimal discomfort.

**Traditional Bronchoscopy** is typically performed by a pulmonologist. In this procedure, a flexible tube called a bronchoscope is passed down the nose or mouth into the trachea, bronchi and larger tubes in the lungs. A bronchoscopy allows the physician to actually see the central regions of the lungs and take a tissue sample for the pathologist to examine. Usually done under local anesthesia with sedation, your healthcare team may do this procedure as an outpatient, so you will not have to spend the night in the hospital. A quick procedure, a bronchoscopy usually takes less than an hour. You may spend several hours "recovering" from the procedure. During this time, the healthcare team will make sure you are awake and not having any problems before you are sent home with your family.

**Electromagnetic Navigation Bronchoscopy™ Procedure**: Also known as ENB™ procedures, Electromagnetic Navigation Bronchoscopy™ procedures are performed by a pulmonologist or thoracic surgeon. ENB™ procedures provide a minimally invasive approach to accessing difficult-to-reach areas of the lung aiding in the diagnosis of lung disease.

Using your CAT scan, Covidien's superDimension™ navigation system with LungGPS™ technology creates a roadmap of your lungs, like a GPS (Global Positioning System) does in a car. That roadmap guides your physician through the airways of your lungs to the nodule. Your physician will insert a bronchoscope through your mouth or nose and into your lungs. With the bronchoscope in place, your physician is able to navigate through your natural airways to the lung nodule. Using tiny instruments, your physician will take a sample of the nodule for testing.

In some cases, small markers may be placed near the lung nodule to help guide a physician delivering follow-up treatment or therapy.

Covidien's LungGPS™ technology used in the superDimension™ navigation system is state-of-the-art, and proven. Ask your doctor if an ENB™ procedure is appropriate for you. Visit the Our Generous Supporters chapter of this guidebook for more information on Covidien's technology.

**Thoracentesis** is performed by an interventional radiologist or pulmonologist. If any of the x-ray procedures show that fluid is present in the chest cavity outside of the lungs, your doctor may insert a thin needle into the chest between the ribs to pull out a sample of the fluid. If you are having trouble breathing because of the amount of fluid in the chest, the doctor may remove more of the fluid to help your breathing. The pathologist will examine the fluid that is removed from the chest.

**Lymph Node Biopsy** is performed by an interventional radiologist or pulmonologist. A lymph node biopsy is done after the initial diagnosis of lung cancer to see if cancer has spread from the lung to the lymph nodes. Lymph node biopsy is an important step in determining the stage of the lung cancer. This procedure can be done in one of three ways: by inserting a needle directly into the lymph node, by using a needle during a bronchoscopy or mediastinoscopy, or by complete removal of the lymph node with surgery. Any of these methods will typically be done on an outpatient basis with local anesthesia. The type of anesthesia and recovery will differ by type of procedure.

**Mediastinoscopy** is performed by a thoracic or general surgeon. For this procedure, you will go to the operating room where you will be given general anesthesia so that you are asleep during the procedure. Your surgeon will place a tube called a mediastinoscope through a small incision in your neck. With the bronchoscopy, the surgeon is able to see inside your lungs; during the mediastinoscopy, the surgeon will be examining the mediastinum (the area between and in front of your lungs). During this procedure, the surgeon can biopsy any lymph nodes or masses seen outside of the lungs. The mediastinoscopy may be done at the same time as a bronchoscopy; if so, both procedures will take less than two hours. If no other procedures are done, a mediastinoscopy usually takes about 45 minutes and may be done on an outpatient basis.

**Video-Assisted Thoracoscopic Surgery (VATS)** is performed by a thoracic surgeon. For the VATS procedure, you will be taken to the operating room and will be given general anesthesia so that you are asleep during the procedure. A thoracoscope is placed into the chest through an incision in the chest wall. A thoracoscope is a camera on the end of flexible tubing that allows your doctor to look into your chest. Your surgeon can then look at the surface of the lung and the chest wall. Your doctor may use the VATS technique to remove some lung cancer tumors. This procedure is less invasive than a thoracotomy and has a shorter recovery time.

**Thoracotomy** is performed by a thoracic surgeon. A thoracotomy is something like a VATS procedure; however, instead of inserting a scope through a small incision, your surgeon will make a larger incision into the chest in order to see the lung directly. In a thoracotomy, a tumor, lung tissue or lymph nodes may be removed. This procedure is done under general anesthesia and you will probably be in the hospital for 3 to 5 days. Your surgeon may elect to do the VATS procedure instead of a thoracotomy.

**What happens to my biopsy and what does it tell my physician?**
When your doctor completes the biopsy, he or she will send the biopsy tissue to

the lab where the pathologist takes a very small slice of the tissue to look at under a microscope. Each type of cell looks very different under a microscope so the pathologist will be able to tell the type of tumor you have and whether it is benign or malignant (cancerous or not).

If the piece of biopsy tissue is large enough, the pathologist may also be able to "grade" the tumor. When the pathologist grades the tumor, he is comparing the tumor cells to normal cells. The tumor grade describes how much the cells from the biopsy tissue resemble normal lung cells. Tumor grades are different for different kinds of cancer, but typically, a lower grade is better. Based on what he sees under the microscope, the pathologist will also determine how fast the tumor may grow and spread.

When your pathologist grades your tumor, he will also send your tissue for molecular testing. Because we know that different types of lung cancer are caused by new or acquired mutations that have different genomic forms, we can use *molecular testing* to identify the specific genomic makeup of the tumor. Knowing the specific genetic form of your tumor may help your team to create a treatment plan that is specific to your tumor.

On tissue biopsies that are larger, the pathologist will also look at the lung tissue around the tumor to see if there are cancer cells outside of the tumor and in the lung tissue. The pathologist prepares a pathology report that includes all of the findings and sends that report to the rest of your healthcare team.

Your healthcare team will use the tumor grade and other findings to begin to develop a treatment plan designed specifically for you. Your doctor will help you understand exactly what the grade of your tumor means and how the grade will help guide your treatment.

## Why does the doctor need to repeat the biopsy?

When you are initially diagnosed the pathologist's first priority is to use your tissue biopsy to determine which specific type of lung cancer you have. This often requires looking at multiple slices of the tumor tissue and applying special stains to the tissue to help with the right diagnosis. The result is often that the tissue is used up and there is nothing left for genomic testing. This happens with 30% to 50% of lung cancer biopsies, especially when they are smaller needle biopsies (1–3).

The more common reason for repeating genomic testing is because the initial tissue sample was only partly genotyped or undergenotyped. Sadly, this happens the majority of the time and typically occurs when you are only tested for *EGFR* and *ALK*, and nothing is found. This could be because tests less sensitive than NGS were used for *EGFR* or *ALK* which may miss a significant number of mutations (4–8). Or another common reason for undergenotyping is because local non-NGS testing for *EGFR* and *ALK* depletes or exhausts your tissue sample and so they cannot test for additional genes even though they may be targetable.

Cancer cells evolve over time, especially when the cancer has been treated. Your cancer one year from diagnosis for example, isn't necessarily the same cancer originally seen under the microscope when you were first diagnosed. The only way to know what the cancer has potentially evolved into is to re-biopsy the tissue and examine it for changes.

Fortunately, there are "liquid biopsy tests" available that use NGS so that you can get complete genomic testing with as simple blood test. We estimate that one of these methods, Guardant360, is likely to find a mutation that drives your cancer in lung adenocarcinoma in all but about ¼ of patients. When you are initially diagnosed there is almost never more than one driver mutation found. Some are targetable and many are not, but if any driving mutation is found then there is no need to repeat an invasive biopsy.

If your cancer has been treated with a targeted therapy but has progressed, a liquid biopsy may be used initially instead of repeating an invasive biopsy. The results typically come back in 10-14 days and if the blood test does not detect the new mutations driving your cancer, then your doctor may recommend a repeat invasive tissue biopsy.

## MOLECULAR TESTING

One of the goals of your treatment is to determine whether your tumor will respond to a particular drug or treatment. Historically, lung cancer was treated based only on type and stage with cytotoxic chemotherapy. Cytotoxic means cell-killing and typically this chemotherapy kills rapidly dividing cells. Chemotherapy may be very effective in some people, but because the cancer cells are not the only rapidly dividing cells, there are often side effects when blood cell producing cells or hair cells (which also rapidly divide) are killed. We are learning that different types of lung cancer have different genomic forms that we can identify through *molecular testing*. Identifying the specific genomic makeup of the tumor may allow your team to tailor your treatment plan to the specific tumor.

The role of molecular testing in lung cancer has grown in the past year. Ask your doctor if molecular testing is available to you. If not, contact us at 1-650-598-2857 to learn how to have your lung cancer tested.

### What is molecular testing?

Molecular testing, also called assays or profiles, can help your treatment team identify specific *biomarkers* that are in your tumor. Molecules contain biomarkers that determine how your cancer will respond to treatment. A biomarker (or biological marker) is a very distinctive substance that indicates a particular disease is present. Biomarkers can be proteins, genes, or other biological substances. A biopsy must be performed to obtain an ideal amount of your tumor tissue for testing. When the tumor is biopsied, your oncologist and pathologist will look for certain biomarkers that have been associated with lung cancer.

The results of these tests determine your distinct 'molecular fingerprint.' Just as no two fingerprints are alike, neither are molecular fingerprints. The information contained in your unique molecular fingerprint gives your oncologist or treating physician insights into how to personalize your lung cancer treatment plan. Each time you have a biopsy, your doctor may order molecular testing on the tissue.

27

When the pathologist identifies specific biomarkers, this may indicate a *genetic mutation* and/or *fusion*. A genetic mutation is anything that changes the structure of a gene. A genetic fusion is a gene that is formed when the genetic material from two previously separate genes are mixed or fused together to form a new cancer-causing gene. We are learning that there are certain genes that can work to produce or suppress lung cancers. When there are changes in the structure (or mutations) of these genes, lung cancer can be the result.

### What specific information is obtained from my molecular testing and how does it determine my personalized treatment?

Different molecular tests are done depending on the laboratory where the tissue is sent. Many major cancer centers at teaching hospitals can perform molecular testing. However, most labs will test the DNA from your tumor in tissue or blood for only *EGFR* mutations and *ALK* fusions, and omit the other five genomic alterations which can be treated with targeted therapies instead of chemotherapy. The seven genes recommended for testing in the national guidelines are found over one third of patients with non-squamous non-small cell lung cancer. [9,10] Many patients tissue biopsy is used up or exhausted with one-at-a time testing for *EGFR* and *ALK*, so that the other five genes (*BRAF, MET, ERBB2 (HER2), RET* and *ROS1*) go untested. Yet 20% or one in five patients with lung adenocarcinoma have one of these other alterations.

# 31% of Lung Adenocarcinoma is Targetable
NCCN Genomic Targets: EGFR, BRAF, MET, ERBB2 (HER2), ALK, ROS1, RET

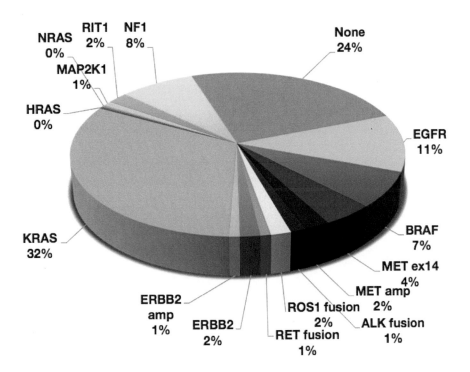

TCGA Nature 2014

This is one reason guidelines recommend that everyone insist on comprehensive genotyping of their tumor with tissue or blood, as with NGS of tissue or blood all seven genomic targets can be tested. [11,12] More and more drug therapies that are targeted or matched to cancers with these and other specific mutations are being developed all the time so we expect new clinical trials and treatment options for lung cancer patients who get NGS testing of their tissue or blood.

- EGFR: The EGFR gene produces a protein called epidermal growth factor receptor. In 10% of patients with non-small cell lung cancer (NSCLC), the EGFR gene is mutated.[8] Nearly 50% of the lung cancers resulting from EGFR mutation happen in people who have never smoked.[9] EGFR mutations are found in about 15% of Caucasians but have about a 40% prevalence in East Asians. The prevalence in Latin Americans and South Asians is intermediate at about 22%.[13]

29

- *KRAS:* The *KRAS* gene is mutated in about 25% of people with NSCLC.[9] There are three drugs that are commonly used to treat lung cancer – gefitinib (Iressa™) and erlotinib (Tarceva®) and afatinib (Gilotrif®). Researchers have found that *EGFR* genomic mutation tumors are sensitive to these *EGFR* inhibitors – that is, the growth of *EGFR* tumors may be slowed by these drugs. On the other hand, tumors with the *KRAS* mutation are resistant to these drugs and they will not work for these tumors. *KRAS* mutations are not targetable so your only option is cytotoxic chemotherapy if mutated.

- *ALK* fusions: In addition to alterations in the *EGFR* or *KRAS* genes, another abnormality called an *ALK* fusion may be the genomic alteration driving your lung cancer. This mutation occurs when two genes (such as *EML4* and *ALK*) become fused into a form that increases the activity of the *ALK* oncogene. The *EML4-ALK* and other *ALK* fusions are found in nearly 5% of patients with non-small cell lung tumors and is highly responsive to a targeted therapy called crizotinib.[9] It is also present in about 10 to 15% of people with non-small cell lung cancer who have never smoked.[9]

- *BRAF:* The fourth identified mutation, *BRAF*, occurs in about 3% of people with lung cancer.[9] Like *KRAS*, this mutation seems to happen most often in patients who are either current smokers or who smoked in the past.

  The *BRAF* mutation produces a protein that transmits signals within a cell to its interior. In a cancer tumor, this signal can cause cells to divide and cancer to grow. About half of the mutations in *BRAF* are now targetable with a *RAF* inhibitor which can block the signal and slow the spread of cancer.[14]

- *MET:* There are several different alterations in the *MET* gene which are responsive to matched therapy. These include point mutations, a deletion of a part of the gene known as exon 14, or amplification where the tumor is driven by extra copies of the *MET* gene even though it is not mutated. All three of these types of alterations are not routinely measured unless comprehensive genomic testing with tissue or blood with NGS is used. This is another reasons we recommend NGS testing, because all three of these alterations in *MET* may respond to crizotinib treatment. About 6% of patients with lung adenocarcinoma have mutations in the *MET* gene, and it occurs with higher frequencies in current or past smokers than in non-smokers.[9,15]

- *ROS1:* ROS1 fusions, like *ALK* fusions, are formed when the *ROS1* gene and a second gene break apart and fuse together with the result of activating the *ROS1* oncogene. These targetable alterations occur in about 2% of lung adenocarcinoma [9] and are targetable with crizotinib.

- *RET: RET* fusions also occur in about 1% [9] of lung adenocarcinomas. Recently these have been shown to be targetable with available matched therapy drugs and exciting new *RET* inhibitors are available in clinical trials.[6]

See the chapter on Targeted Therapies for more information on the role of molecular testing and treatment decisions.

## Blood-based proteomic testing

If genetic sequencing is similar to the "script" of biology, then proteomics (the study of proteins) is the live video capturing biology in action. One of the advantages of proteomics is that cancer patient subgroups have been identified based on specific protein signatures expressed by the tumor cells or the patient's immune response to the tumor. These protein signatures can be detected in the patient's blood (no tissue biopsy) and can be used to help inform the patient's treatment plan.

Biodesix Inc., is a molecular diagnostics company advancing the development of innovative blood-based tests in oncology for precision medicine. VeriStrat® is a commercially available serum proteomic test, used for both prognosis and diagnosis in advanced NSCLC. The company provides physicians with diagnostic tests for earlier disease detection, more accurate diagnosis, disease monitoring and better therapeutic guidance, which may lead to improved patient outcomes. **Visit www.biodesix.com**

## Future of molecular testing

Other genetic biomarkers and mutations that are currently being studied could provide additional specific treatments for non-small cell lung cancer. Molecular testing ensures the right drug for the right patient at the right time. Be sure to speak with your oncologist about molecular testing. If you still have questions on how to obtain molecular testing, contact us at 1-650-598-2857.

## Next-Generation Sequencing

Genomic testing or profiling identifies the underlying DNA alterations that are driving the tumor's growth. This information may help physicians understand which targeted treatment options are available for a patient based on their tumor's unique genomic profile. A new technology called next-generation sequencing (NGS) is often referenced in relation to molecular or genomic testing for lung cancer. NGS is a tool for sequencing large amounts of DNA accurately in a short period of time, but it can be applied in many different ways.

Standard genomic testing examines only one or a limited set of cancer-related genes and does not provide a complete picture. Some tests may use NGS to look for a few types of alterations in predetermined "hotspot" regions within genes where alterations more commonly occur. However, tumors often contain multiple alterations that would be missed by these more narrowly focused genomic tests, limiting potential treatment options.

In fact, national guidelines for non-small cell lung cancer recommend comprehensive NGS testing so that no potentially treatable genomic alterations are overlooked. For example, hotspot testing for the most common mutations in the *EGFR* gene would still miss 1/6 of the *EGFR* mutations that occur.[5]

A comprehensive genomic profiling test uses NGS to look at all of the cancer-related genes in a single sample of tumor tissue and detects all types of alterations. This approach provides the information your physician needs in one single test to help guide a tailored treatment approach using targeted therapies. You and your doctor can use the results from a comprehensive genomic profile to discuss possible treatment options, including FDA-approved targeted therapies or novel targeted treatments under development in clinical trials.

Comprehensive genomic profiling is a relatively new treatment tool and not yet covered by all insurance carriers in the U.S., but coverage may be appealed on a case-by-case basis and financial assistance may be available. We will keep you updated on comprehensive genomic profiling as new information comes available. In the meantime, if you would like comprehensive genomic profiling performed on your lung cancer tumor, you can find more information and a discussion guide for you and your physician at www.dontguesstestlungcancer.com or call ALCF at 1-650-598-2857.

There are three laboratories that we recommend you consider for comprehensive genomic profiling: Caris Life Sciences, Foundation Medicine and Guardant Health. Caris requires a tissue biopsy for testing, Foundation requires either tissue or a blood sample, and Guardant Health requires only a blood sample.

Caris Life Sciences' evidence-guided tumor profiling service, Caris Molecular Intelligence™, provides oncologists with the most potentially clinically actionable treatment options available to personalize cancer care today. Using a variety of advanced and validated technologies, which assess relevant biological changes in each patient's tumor, Caris Molecular Intelligence correlates biomarker data generated from a tumor with biomarker-drug associations supported by evidence in the relevant clinical literature. To learn more about Caris Molecular Intelligence™ visit their website at www.CarisLifeSciences.com.

Foundation Medicine offers FoundationOne, a comprehensive genomic profiling test that helps physicians make treatment decisions for patients with cancer by identifying the molecular growth drivers of their cancers and helping oncologists match them with relevant targeted therapeutic options or clinical trials. To learn more about Foundation Medicine, visit www.foundationmedicine.com. To learn more about the Foundation One test and for other resources to help you understand the testing process, visit www.mycancerisunique.com.

Guardant Health, the world's leader in liquid biopsies, offers a comprehensive genomic test called Guardant360. This non-invasive blood biopsy can detect all of the genomic alterations found in lung cancer that are relevant for targeted therapies. Requiring just two vials of blood, Guardant360 helps oncologists provide personalized cancer care by matching patients to FDA-approved therapies as well as clinical trials. To learn more about the most validated and comprehensive blood based test on the market visit www.guardanthealth.com/guardant360

### How is my tumor tissue for molecular testing obtained?

One of your doctors will do a biopsy to get a tissue sample from your tumor. Cancer diagnosis always begins with a tissue biopsy so that a pathologist can determine which type of cancer you have. Biopsies can be performed in a number of ways. It is important to get a big enough piece of tumor tissue to do molecular testing. Fine needle aspiration (FNA) biopsy may not provide enough tissue for molecular testing, so your oncologist may recommend one of the following methods for biopsy.

- Core needle biopsy performed by an interventional radiologist
- Bronchoscopy performed by a pulmonologist
- Lymph node biopsy performed by an interventional radiologist or pulmonologist
- Mediastinoscopy performed by a thoracic or general surgeon
- Computed tomography (CT), fluoroscopy, ultrasound, or MRI-guided core needle biopsy performed by an interventional radiologist or pulmonologist
- Video-assisted thoracoscopic surgery performed by a thoracic surgeon
- Electromagnetic Navigation Bronchoscopy™ procedure performed by a pulmonologist or thoracic surgeon

### What if the biopsy does not produce enough tissue to test for all the known genetic mutations?

There are seven genes whose alterations cause non-small cell lung cancer (NSCLC), that currently have an FDA approved drug associated with them. Patients with these alterations comprise almost 85% of lung cancers (small cell lung cancer incidence has gradually declined to < 15 of lung cancers). (ref Govindan R: Changing Epidemiology of Small-Cell Lung Cancer in the United States Over the Last 30 Years: Analysis of the

Surveillance, Epidemiologic, and End Results Database. J Clin Oncol 24:4539–4544, 2006 ) Recent National Comprehensive Cancer Network guidelines (ref www.nccn.org) strongly recommend broad molecular profiling to cover all seven genomic targets in NSCLC: (*EGFR, ALK, ROS1, BRAF, MET, RET* and *HER2*) as these have matched therapy treatments which produce responses 2-3 times higher than chemotherapy alone. If the doctor does not get enough tissue to test for all genetic markers, NCCN guidelines recommend blood (plasma) testing (a "liquid biopsy") when a repeat invasive tissue biopsy is infeasible (please note these blood biopsies although on the brink of being FDA approved, they are currently not). (ref NCCN).

### Where will my tissue be tested?

A Clinical Laboratory Improvement Amendments certified laboratory, most commonly referred to as a CLIA certified laboratory, will usually test the tumor tissue. If your hospital does not have a lab that offers the molecular testing, your oncologist will ask that the tissue be sent to another lab.

### How long does it take to get my results?

Your oncologist will get the results of the molecular testing within 3 to 10 business days. Your oncologist may call you with the results or discuss them with you at your next appointment. Either way, your oncologist will discuss the results and treatment options that may be appropriate for you based on those results.

## OTHER DIAGNOSTIC TESTS

### Pulmonary Function Test (PFT)

The PFT is a breathing test to determine how well your lungs are working. This non-painful test may be performed in your pulmonologist's office or in the hospital on an outpatient basis.

### Pulse Oximetry (Pulse Ox)

One of the common symptoms you might experience with lung cancer is shortness of breath. Your team may use a device called a pulse oximeter to measure the level of oxygen in your blood. The pulse oximeter is placed on your fingertip for a minute. A low level of oxygen in your blood may prompt your doctor to order extra oxygen for you during your illness.

## High Altitude Simulation Test (HAST)

The High Altitude Simulation Test (HAST) is a test your doctor may use to find out if you will need oxygen when you fly or travel to a high altitude city or country. You may also hear HAST called a "hypoxia altitude simulation test." When you fly or are at a high altitude, you may be at risk for cardiopulmonary (heart or lung) problems due to the lower oxygen available. During the HAST exam, your doctor will take your blood pressure, pulse and respiratory rate before the test begins and while you are breathing your normal air mixture. The doctor may also connect you to a cardiac monitor that will allow the team to monitor your heart rhythm. After those initial measurements, you will breathe air that contains a lower percentage of oxygen than you may be used to. During the 20 to 30 minutes of the test, your doctor will monitor you for any significant symptoms you have while breathing the air with lower oxygen. If you have symptoms during the test, the doctor will test you again while giving you oxygen to ensure that the additional oxygen will prevent the symptoms. The doctor doing the test will send results of the HAST to your oncologist and pulmonologist.

## Complete Blood Count (CBC)

Chemotherapy and radiation therapy can temporarily affect the cells of the bone marrow that produce normal blood cells, so your healthcare team will want to keep track of this important test before and during treatment. A CBC can also alert your doctor to certain abnormalities in the blood that may indicate problems with the function of your kidneys or liver. Your doctor will order a CBC on a regular basis to determine if your blood has the correct number and types of cells.

## Sputum Cytology

For the sputum cytology test, a member of your healthcare team will ask you to cough up a sample of mucus (sputum) from as deep in your lungs as possible. Lung cancer cells can shed into the airway and mix with mucus there. When you produce a sputum sample, the cytologist or pathologist will examine the sputum looking for normal or abnormal cells. Cytology is the study of cells and a cytologist is a scientist who studies the identification of cancer cells.

## DIAGNOSIS TIMELINE

### How long should I expect to wait for results and, ultimately, a diagnosis?

The timeline for the diagnosis of lung cancer may vary greatly based on who your physician is, the institution where you are being treated, your treatment plan and possible other diagnostic tests that may need to be performed. Following is a timeline that ALCF would be pleased to see as the standard of care for the diagnosis of lung cancer.

It is important to work with an oncologist who specializes in lung cancer and that you have a multidisciplinary team to manage your cancer journey. Ask your doctor to refer you to a lung cancer specialist or call ALCF for referrals at 1-650-598-2857.

Following an x-ray that shows a suspicious spot on the lung, you should get a CT scan. If the CT scan shows a spot, your doctor will schedule a biopsy. Following the biopsy, depending on the type of lung cancer found in your tumor, your doctor might want to perform molecular testing.

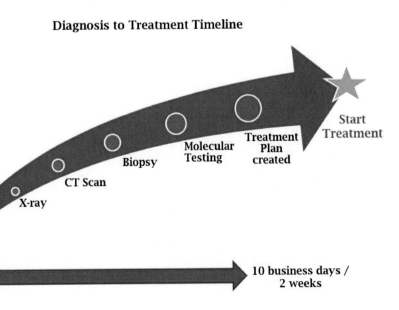

**Diagnosis to Treatment Timeline**

X-ray
CT Scan
Biopsy
Molecular Testing
Treatment Plan created
Start Treatment

10 business days / 2 weeks

If your oncologist recommends infusion (in the vein) chemotherapy and you decide to have an intravenous port inserted, your team will schedule and perform this procedure. Depending on the treatment recommended by your oncologist, access to the chemotherapy drugs may take time. In the ideal circumstances, the time from identification of a possible tumor to treatment may take up to two weeks. This timeline may vary depending on the availability of services in your area—but this timeline should be the goal for your treatment team.

## My doctor says I have lung cancer. What happens next?

Your family doctor or the doctor who helped diagnose the lung cancer will refer you to an oncologist who will work with you to design your treatment plan. You may also have a radiation oncologist if you will be receiving radiation treatments for the cancer.

Your healthcare team may also consist of many other people from many different specialties whose job it is to help you understand your disease and make your treatments as comfortable as possible.

## Can I get a second opinion?

Before starting treatment, you may want a second opinion about your diagnosis and treatment plan. Many insurance companies cover the cost of a second opinion if you or your doctor requests it. There are many ways to find a doctor for a second opinion. The best way is to have your doctor refer you to someone he or she trusts. If your doctor refers you, the time to get an appointment may be much shorter. You can also get names of physicians and medical centers specializing in lung cancer by contacting ALCF at 1-650-598-2857, calling or writing a local or state medical society, talking to social workers at your local hospital, or asking at a nearby medical school for names of specialists they recommend. Your nearest cancer center or cancer support group may also be excellent sources of names for second opinions.

Before going to see another doctor for a second opinion, be sure to collect all your medical records, including x-rays and pathology reports, to take with you. In some cases, you may be able to have the hospital or your doctor send your records directly to the doctor you will be seeing. Be patient since this process is not always smooth. Ask your doctor if a delay for a second opinion will have a negative impact on your health. In most cases, a delay of less than two weeks will make very little difference in the effectiveness of your treatment plan. Be sure to check with your insurance company about expenses they will cover if you must travel to another city for a second opinion. Some companies will cover all or part of this expense.

### What is the difference between a community cancer center and an academic medical center?

Depending on the treatment prescribed by your oncologist and the options available in your community, you may receive your treatment in a number of settings. First, you may have appointments in your oncologist's office located in a medical office building or community cancer center. The oncologist's office may have a laboratory in the office; this will mean that most lab tests can be done without having to go to another office. Your oncologist may also have an infusion center in his or her office where you will be able to receive chemotherapy treatments.

Second, you may have access to a community cancer center where you can receive most of the care you will need during your treatment. In 2007, the National Cancer Institute (NCI) began the Community Cancer Center Program providing funding to community cancer centers around the country.[10] It is likely that there is a cancer center close to you where the goal is to provide high quality care while advancing cancer research efforts. Many cancer centers are associated with hospitals where you can easily receive your laboratory tests, diagnostic tests and procedures, radiation and chemotherapy treatments and surgical procedures. In addition, most cancer centers also have extensive social service, financial counseling, and other support services you may need during your treatment course.

Finally, you may live close to an academic medical center that is associated with a variety of healthcare schools. If you do have access to an academic center, you may be able to receive more specialized treatment using technologies that are more advanced. Often, an academic medical center will have available innovative treatments that may not be available in a community hospital. Be aware that since these academic centers are associated with medical, nursing and other healthcare schools, your treatment team will likely include students and researchers learning new skills and conducting clinical trials. An academic medical center will also have extensive social service, financial counseling, and other support services you may need during your treatment course.

Depending on the type of facilities near you, the resources available may be very different. It is important to find a cancer center that has the resources you need to support you during your cancer treatment. Where you receive your care is as important as finding an oncologist who specializes in treating lung cancer. We are here to help—contact ALCF at 1-650-598-2857 for a referral to a cancer center.

## MULTIDISCIPLINARY HEALTHCARE TEAM

A multidisciplinary team is ideal! The following is a list of medical professionals you may have on your healthcare team. Some of these people may have different titles, and the same person may fill some of these roles, but you should have access to these services:

**Medical Oncologist:** A medical oncologist is a physician who treats cancer using medications and chemotherapy drugs.

**Radiation Oncologist:** A radiation oncologist is a physician who uses x-rays and special radiology procedures in cancer diagnosis and treatment. This includes x-rays, CT scans, MRI, and PET scans.

**Thoracic Surgeon:** A thoracic surgeon is a physician who specializes in the surgical treatment of cancer and other diseases of the chest.

**Pulmonologist:** A pulmonologist is a physician who specializes in the evaluation and treatment of lung problems.

**Pathologist:** A pathologist is a physician who analyzes tumor tissues removed by biopsy or surgery in order to diagnose and stage cancer and other diseases.

**RN Navigator:** An RN Navigator is a registered nurse who will help you and your family by offering education, support and coordination of services in the process of diagnosis and treatment of cancer.

**Chemotherapy Nurse:** A chemotherapy nurse is a registered nurse who specializes in the delivery of chemotherapy and other cancer treatments, helping you deal with any side effects and placing IVs for infusions.

**Research Nurse:** A research nurse is a registered nurse who administers and provides nursing care if you are involved in clinical trials.

**Symptom Management Care Coordinator:** A symptom management care coordinator is a registered nurse or physician who will help you manage symptoms associated with disease and treatment of cancer.

**Radiation Technician:** A radiation technician is a licensed professional who will guide you through radiation treatments, inject dyes or contrast for radiation tests, and care for you during radiation treatments.

**Social Worker:** A social worker is a licensed professional who will be available to assist you and your family with supportive counseling and community resources.

**Registered Dietitian:** A registered dietitian is a licensed professional who will help you develop a nutritional plan based on your specific needs.

**Bonnie J. Addario Lung Cancer Foundation (ALCF):** ALCF is one of the largest patient-founded, patient-focused, and patient-driven philanthropies devoted exclusively to eradicating lung cancer through research, early detection, education, and treatment. The Foundation is available to assist you along your cancer journey. Simply call us at 1-650-598-2857.

**What should I do if a multi-disciplinary team is not readily available?**

If you live in an area far from a cancer center or major medical center, you may want to travel to have a second opinion or to access more resources. A medical oncologist at a major medical center may be willing to work with your local oncologist to ensure that you get the most advanced care as possible at your local hospital or clinic. If you are unable to travel to a cancer center or major medical center, ask your local oncologist for help identifying the resources you need to manage your treatment course. We are here to help; feel free to contact us at ALCF at 1-650-598-2857 for information on local resources.

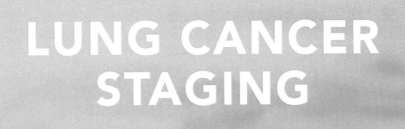

*The Patient Education Handbook was and still is my go to for information. It's been five years since I was diagnosed and I still refer back to the handbook for information.*

*—Kimberly Buchmeier, survivor*

# LUNG CANCER STAGING

In addition to grading the tumor, your healthcare team will also stage your lung cancer.

**What does the stage of my lung cancer mean?**
The stage of your lung cancer tells your oncologist the size of the primary tumor, the number of lymph nodes with cancer cells in them, and if the cancer has spread to other organs. Knowing the stage of the lung cancer is critical because the stage of lung cancer will help you and your oncologist determine the types of treatment that will be most effective for you.

> Questions for your physician about staging your lung cancer:
> - What stage is my lung cancer and what does that mean for me?
> - Has the cancer spread from my lung to other parts of my body?
> - Will I need more tests before deciding which treatments to take?

You may be familiar with the traditional staging of lung cancer in which your oncologist may describe the stages as Stage I, II, III or IV. In this staging, the higher number indicates lung cancer that is more extensive. Oncologists also use the TNM system as a way to determine the stage of the lung cancer.

## T, N, M Lung Cancer Staging

The TNM staging system was developed by the American Joint Committee on Cancer (AJCC) and the International Union Against Cancer (UICC). Since the development of this system, it has become one of the most commonly used staging systems for cancer. Your oncologist will use the TNM classification system to stage your cancer based on standard criteria.

According to the 2010 definitions of staging, the letters T, N and M, identify three major pieces of information used for tumor staging:

- T = describes the size of the primary tumor
- N = describes the number of lymph nodes with cancer cells in them
- M = describes the presence of metastatic tumors in distant organs

If your team uses this staging, your doctor might describe the stage of your lung cancer, for example, as T1, N1, M0. This designation would mean that the primary tumor has been identified but is relatively small (T1). There are lymph nodes involved (N1), but the cancer has not spread to other organs (M0).

We understand that the following information may be difficult to understand. To help you understand the staging process, visit the National Cancer Institute website for pictures of each stage of disease. Their website address is http://www.cancer.gov/cancertopics/pdq/treatment/non-small-cell-lung/Patient/page2.

**Stage I, II, III, IV Lung Cancer Staging[11]**

**Stage 0 or Carcinoma in Situ:** If the oncologist says that you have Stage 0, this means that your doctor found abnormal cells in your airway, often with a sputum cytology test. These cells may grow and invade the lung.

**Stage I:** If your oncologist says your lung cancer is Stage I, it means that a tumor has been found in one lung only and there is no cancer found in the lymph nodes.

## Staging chart for Stage I:

| Stages 0 to I of lung cancer | TNM (Tumor, Nodes, Metastasis) | Definition |
|---|---|---|
| Occult carcinoma | TX, N0, M0 | TX = Primary tumour cannot be assessed, or tumour proven by the presence of malignant cells in sputum or bronchial washings but not visualized by imaging or bronchoscopy.<br><br>N0 = No regional lymph node metastasis<br><br>M0 = No distant metastasis |
| 0 | Tis, N0, M0 | Tis = Carcinoma in situ<br><br>N0 = No regional lymph node metastasis<br><br>M0 = No distant metastasis |
| IA | T1a, N0, M0<br><br>T1b, N0, M0 | T1a = Tumour ≤2 cm in greatest dimension<br><br>T1b = Tumour >2 cm but ≤3 in greatest dimension<br><br>N0 = No regional lymph node metastasis<br><br>M0 = No distant metastasis |
| IB | T2a, N0, M0 | T2a = Tumour >3 cm but ≤5 cm in greatest dimension<br><br>N0 = No regional lymph node metastasis<br><br>M0 = No distant metastasis |

Provided courtesy of the International Association for the Study of Lung Cancer.[11]

**Stage II:** Stage II lung cancer means that your doctor has found cancer in one lung only and there may be lymph node involvement on the same side as the lung cancer. In Stage II cancer, the cancer is not found in the lymph nodes in the mediastinum. The mediastinum is the area between the lungs from the breastbone and the spinal column.

Stage chart for Stage II:

| Stage II of lung cancer | TNM (Tumor, Nodes, metastasis) | Definition |
|---|---|---|
| IIA | T1a, N1, M0 | T1a = Tumour ≤2 cm in greatest dimension |
| | T1b, N1, M0 | T1b = Tumour >2 cm but ≤3 cm in greatest dimension |
| | T2a, N1, M0 | T2a = Tumour >3 cm but ≤5 cm in greatest dimension |
| | | N1 = metastasis in ipsilateral peribronchial and/or ipsilateral hilar lymph nodes and intrapulmonary nodes, including involvement by direct extension |
| | | M0 = No distant metastasis |
| | T2b, N0, M0 | T2b = Tumour >5 cm but ≤7 cm in greatest dimension |
| | | N0 = No regional lymph node metastasis |
| | | M0 = No distant metastasis |

Provided courtesy of the International Association for the Study of Lung Cancer.[11]

| Stage II of lung cancer | TNM (Tumor, Nodes, metastasis) | Definition |
|---|---|---|
| IIB | T2b, N1, M0 | T2b = Tumour >5 cm but ≤7 cm in greatest dimension<br><br>N1 = metastasis in ipsilateral peribronchial and/or ipsilateral hilar lymph nodes and intrapulmonary nodes, including involvement by direct extension<br><br>M0 = No distant metastasis |
| | T3, N0, M0 | T3 = Tumour >7 cm or one that directly invades any of the following: chest wall (including superior sulcus tumours), diaphragm, phrenic nerve, mediastinal pleura, parietal pericardium; or tumour in the main bronchus less than 2 cm distal to the carina but without involvement of the carina; or associated atelectasis or obstructive pneumonitis of the entire lung or separate tumour nodule(s) in the same lobe as the primary.<br><br>N0 = No regional lymph node metastasis<br><br>M0 = No distant metastasis |

Provided courtesy of the International Association for the Study of Lung Cancer.[11]

**Stage IIIA:** Stage IIIA lung cancer means that there may be one or more tumors in the same lobe of the lung. In this stage, the cancer has also spread to the lymph nodes on the same side of the lung as the cancer or to where the trachea joins the bronchus, the chest wall, or the lining around the lung.

Staging chart for Stage IIIA:

| Stage IIIA of lung cancer | TNM (Tumor, Nodes, Metastasis) | Definition |
|---|---|---|
| IIIA | T1a, N2, M0 | T1a = Tumour ≤2 cm in greatest dimension |
| | T1b, N2, M0 | T1b = Tumour >2 cm but ≤3 cm in greatest dimension |
| | T2a, N2, M0 | T2a = Tumour >3 cm but ≤5 cm in greatest dimension |
| | T2b, N2, M0 | T2b = Tumour >5 cm but ≤7 cm in greatest dimension |
| | | N2 = Metastasis in ipsilateral mediastinal and/or subcarinal lymph node(s) |
| | | M0 = No distant metastasis |

| Stage IIIA of lung cancer | TNM (Tumor, Nodes, Metastasis) | Definition |
|---|---|---|
| | T3, N1, M0 | T3 = Tumour >7 cm or one that directly invades any of the following: chest wall (including superior sulcus tumours), diaphragm, phrenic nerve, mediastinal pleura, parietal pericardium; or tumour in the main bronchus less than 2 cm distal to the carina but without involvement of the carina; or associated atelectasis or obstructive pneumonitis of the entire lung or separate tumour nodule(s) in the same lobe as the primary.<br><br>N1 = Metastasis in ipsilateral peribronchial and/or ipsilateral hilar lymph nodes and intrapulmonary nodes, including involvement by direct extension<br><br>M0 = No distant metastasis. |
| | T3, N2, M0 | T3 = Tumour >7 cm or one that directly invades any of the following: chest wall (including superior sulcus tumours), diaphragm, phrenic nerve, mediastinal pleura, parietal pericardium; or tumour in the main bronchus less than 2 cm distal to the carina but without involvement of the carina; or associated atelectasis or obstructive pneumonitis of the entire lung or separate tumour nodule(s) in the same lobe as the primary.<br><br>N2 = Metastasis in ipsilateral mediastinal and/or subcarinal lymph node(s)<br><br>M0 = No distant metastasis |
| | T4, N0, M0 | T4 = Tumour of any size that invades any of the following: mediastinum, heart, great vessels, trachea, recurrent laryngeal nerve, oesophagus, vertebral body, carina; separate tumour nodule(s) in a different ipsilateral lobe to that of the primary.<br><br>N0 = No regional lymph node metastasis<br><br>M0 = No distant metastasis |

51

| Stage IIIA of lung cancer | TNM (Tumor, Nodes, metastasis) | Definition |
|---|---|---|
| | T4, N1, M0 | T4 = Tumour of any size that invades any of the following: mediastinum, heart, great vessels, trachea, recurrent laryngeal nerve, oesophagus, vertebral body, carina; separate tumour nodule(s) in a different ipsilateral lobe to that of the primary.<br><br>N1 = Metastasis in ipsilateral peribronchial and/or ipsilateral hilar lymph nodes and intrapulmonary nodes, including involvement by direct extension<br><br>M0 = No distant metastasis |

Provided courtesy of the International Association for the Study of Lung Cancer.[11]

**Stage IIIB:** In Stage IIIB lung cancer, there may be separate tumors in any of the lobes of the lung and the cancer may have spread to the chest wall, diaphragm, lining of the lung or chest wall, lining of the heart or the heart, major blood vessels that lead to or from the heart, esophagus, sternum, or spine.

Staging chart for Stage IIIB:

| Stage IIIB of lung cancer | TNM (Tumor, Nodes, Metastasis) | Definition |
|---|---|---|
| IIIB | T4, N2, M0 | TX = Primary tumour cannot be assessed, or tumour proven by the presence of malignant cells in sputum or bronchial washings but not visualized by imaging or bronchoscopy. N0 = No regional lymph node metastasis M0 = No distant metastasis |
| | Any T, N3, M0 | Any T N3 = Metastasis in contralateral mediastinal, contralateral hilar, ipsilateral or contralateral scalene, or supraclavicular lymph node(s) M0 = No distant metastasis |

Provided courtesy of the International Association for the Study of Lung Cancer.[11]

**Stage IV:** In Stage IV lung cancer, there are one or more tumors in both lungs and cancer may be found in the fluid around the lung. The cancer may have spread through to other organs of the body, often the brain, liver, or the bones.

Staging chart for Stage IV:

| Stage IV of lung cancer | TNM (Tumor, Nodes, Metastasis) | Definition |
|---|---|---|
| IV | Any T, Any N, M1 | Any T<br><br>Any N<br><br>• NX = Regional lymph nodes cannot be assessed<br><br>• N0 = No regional lymph node metastasis<br><br>• N1 = Metastasis in ipsilateral peribronchial and/or ipsilateral hilar lymph nodes and intrapulmonary nodes, including involvement by direct extension<br><br>• N2 = Metastasis in ipsilateral mediastinal and/or subcarinal lymph node(s)<br><br>• N3 = Metastasis in contralateral mediastinal, contralateral hilar, ipsilateral or contralateral scalene, or supraclavicular lymph node(s)<br><br>M1 = Distant Metastasis |

Provided courtesy of the International Association for the Study of Lung Cancer.[11]

While staging is a useful classification, it is important to remember that you must discuss these stages with your healthcare team who will help you understand what the stage means in the context of your specific diagnosis and treatment plan.

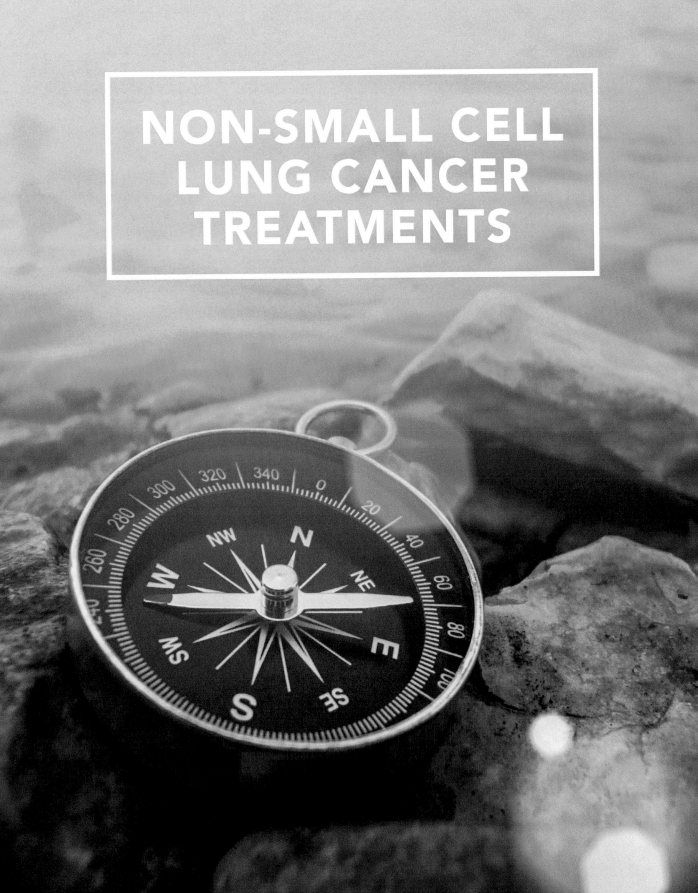

# NON-SMALL CELL LUNG CANCER TREATMENTS

GET INFORMED

**AT THE**

## PATIENT PORTAL

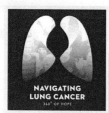

# SIGN UP!!!

## www.lungcancerfoundation.org/patients/portal/

Consider signing up for our Patient Portal where we bring you information customized to your disease and provide you with additional members-only features such as direct, live chat access to the foundation.

This PORTAL is your home on the web to learn about the latest news affecting you, lung cancer patients, and get support from stories shared by other patients, and maybe tell your own.

We are here for you! If you have questions about information you find, navigating the complex path of cancer treatment, or anything else, please don't hesitate to get in touch with us. Your message will be delivered directly to Danielle Hicks (Director of Patient Services and Programs), Michele Zeh (Patient Navigation and Services Coordinator), and Guneet Walia, PhD (Director of Research and Medical Affairs).

If you are ROS1-positive, the portal a section dedicated to ROS1ers.
http://www.lungcancerfoundation.org/patients/ros1/

# NON-SMALL CELL LUNG CANCER – TREATMENTS

## OVERVIEW

After you are diagnosed with lung cancer, your next question is sure to be "What can be done to treat the cancer?" Your individual treatment plan will depend on the type of lung cancer, its stage and your overall health. As you begin to plan your treatment with your healthcare team, it is important that you keep a list of questions you have. This can be a confusing time so remember to write everything down as you discuss your treatment plan with the team.

Possible treatments for lung cancer include surgery, chemotherapy, radiation therapy, targeted therapy or a combination of these.

Lung cancer treatments fall into two categories:

- Local therapy: Surgery and radiation therapy are *local therapies*. They remove or destroy

Questions for your physician regarding lung cancer treatments:

- What are my treatment choices?
- What is the goal of my treatment (curative, stable disease, palliative or symptom management)?
- Will I have more than one type of treatment?
- What are the expected benefits of each type of treatment?
- How will treatment affect my normal activities and daily life?
- What can we do to control the side effects?
- Are there other treatment options available to me?
- Are there any clinical trials available to me?
- What can I do to prepare for treatment?
- Will I need to be hospitalized? If so, for how long?
- What is the cost of treatment? Will my insurance cover the cost?
- Do I have time to seek a 2nd opinion or to think about my treatment options? If so, how long before I need to start treatment?

cancer tumors in the lungs. If lung cancer has spread to other parts of the body, such as other organs or bones, your doctor may use one of these local therapies to control the disease in those specific areas as well.

- Systemic therapy: Chemotherapy and targeted therapies are *systemic therapies*. These drugs enter the bloodstream to destroy or control cancer everywhere in the body. Systemic therapy is taken by mouth or given through a vein in the arm or a port that is inserted in your chest (intravenous).

| Questions for your physician about surgery: |
| --- |
| • What type of surgery do you recommend? |
| • How long will I be in the hospital? |
| • What side effects should I expect? |
| • Will I feel pain? If so, how will it be controlled? |
| • When can I get back to my normal activities? |

## SURGERY FOR THE TREATMENT OF NSCLC

Surgery may be effective for treatment of stages I - III in non-small cell lung cancer.

### When is surgery used to treat lung cancer?

If your NSCLC tumor has not spread to other tissues outside of the lungs, your oncologist may recommend surgery to remove the tumor. Surgery may be the first type of treatment you receive, or your oncologist may recommend other non-surgical treatments first. In some cases, chemotherapy or radiation will be used first to shrink the cancer tumor before surgery. The specific order of treatment depends on the size of the cancer tumor and whether the cancer has spread outside of the lungs.

The tissue that is removed from the lung (specimen) is sent to the pathologist who will look at the edges (or

> Ask your oncologist for a referral to a thoracic surgeon to assist with decisions involving surgery and to perform major surgical procedures on your lung.

margins) of the specimen to see if the tumor has been completely removed. If there are tumor cells at the margin, it may mean that the entire tumor was not removed. These results will determine treatment following surgery.

**What types of surgery might be used to treat me?**

The following are types of surgery for lung cancer:

**To remove a small portion of the lung:**

*Wedge Resection*: In wedge resection, your surgeon will remove a small portion of the lung that contains the tumor. For stage I and II tumors, your surgeon may elect to use VATS, thoracotomy, or the *da Vinci®* surgical system.

*Segmental Resection or Segmentectomy*: In a segemental resection, your surgeon will remove a slightly larger portion of tissue than with a wedge resection but not the whole lobe.

**To remove a lobe of the lung:**

*Sleeve Resection*: In a sleeve resection, the surgeon will try to keep as much of the lung as possible by removing only the lobe (part of lung) with a cancerous tumor. In this surgery, the surgeon will remove the lobe with the cancerous tumor and part of the bronchus (air passage); the lobe of the lung that is left is connected to the remaining bronchus.

*Lobectomy*: In a lobectomy, your surgeon will remove an entire lobe of the lung.

To remove the entire lung:

*Pneumonectomy*: In a pneumonectomy, your surgeon will remove the entire lung.

Sleeve resections and pneumonectomy are used when the lung cancer tumor is larger and closer to the middle of the chest. A lobectomy is used when the lung cancer tumor is more peripherally located (away from the center of the chest).

To remove lymph nodes:

*Lymph Node Dissection or Lymphadenectomy*: During a lymph node dissection, your surgeon will remove several lymph nodes around your tumor to determine if any cancer cells are outside of your lungs. This will help your oncologist determine the stage of the lung cancer and the most appropriate treatment plan. If the pathologist finds cancer cells in the lymph nodes, you may receive chemotherapy after surgery to kill those cells.

### Treatment of Pneumothorax or Recurrent Pleural Effusion

A pneumothorax is a collection of air in the space that separates your lung from your chest wall. When this happens, part of your lung may collapse making it difficult for you to breathe. A pleural effusion happens when fluid collects in the pleural layers that surround the lungs. This condition can also cause difficulty breathing. A pleurodesis is a chemical or surgical procedure that may be done to prevent these conditions from *recurring* (happening another time).

Your oncologist may do a chemical pleurodesis by injecting a drug into the pleural space around the lungs through a drain or tube in your chest. The drug acts as an irritant that closes the pleural space and prevents fluid from entering the space.

You will be given a local anesthetic that will numb the area on your chest where the tube enters. You may also be given a drug to relax you before the procedure starts.

A surgical pleurodesis is done by making an incision into your chest and rubbing the pleural layers with a rough pad to irritate the pleural lining. Your surgeon may also remove some of the parietal tissue. Either of these surgical procedures will be done under anesthesia.

**Advantages of surgical removal of a lung tumor:**

- If the margins of the tumor and lymph nodes outside of the lung do not contain cancer cells, surgery can be a cure for lung cancer.
- Because the surgeon removes all or most of the tumor, the size of the tumor tissue will be large enough for molecular testing and to stage the tumor. The combination of accurate staging and molecular testing will enable your oncologist to develop an individualized treatment plan specific to your type of lung cancer.
- Your surgeon can do a pleurodesis to prevent fluid from collecting between the lung and its lining.

**Disadvantages of surgical removal of a lung tumor:**

- Long recovery time
- Not all the cancer may be removed
- Risks associated with invasive surgery

**What to expect during and after surgery:**

- The surgeon will do the surgery procedure in the operating room.
- An anesthesiologist will use general anesthesia to put you to sleep for the for the procedure.

- You will remain in the hospital for about one week for recovery.
- Your doctor may order an epidural for pain control and other drugs to control pain.
- Your surgeon may insert a chest tube to drain any fluid that might collect after surgery.
- The respiratory therapist will teach you some breathing and strengthening
- exercises to help you recover more quickly after surgery.
- Your doctor may prescribe an inhaler filled with medicine to help you if you
- have trouble breathing.

**Possible side effects of a surgical procedure:**

- You may have pain from the surgery or chest tube incision; be sure to ask for pain medicine <u>before</u> your pain is severe. Controlling pain will be a large part of your recovery.
- You may experience some neuralgia (numbness) on the side of your chest where you had surgery.
- If fluid builds up around the lungs, you might develop a condition called a pleural effusion. This condition may cause you to have trouble breathing. Call your doctor if you notice shortness of breath that does not go away when you rest.
- The anesthesiologist will insert a tube into your throat during surgery to help you breathe during the procedure. This tube may injure one or both of your vocal cords resulting in hoarseness or difficulty speaking.
- Depending on the extent of the surgery, you may have weeks of recovery time following surgery.
- Women may want to avoid wearing a bra for a week or two after surgery because of pain and discomfort around the ribs.

- There are other possible side effects. Your surgeon and the surgical team will discuss the benefits and risks of surgery and anesthesia prior to surgery. Be sure to ask questions.

**Tips for recovering from surgery – A patient's perspective**
After any surgery for lung cancer, you may have side effects because of the surgery. I know because I have been there. Your healthcare team will be able to tell you many things you can do to recover after surgery, but there are some things only another patient can tell you. A few things I have learned in my own journey that may help you as you recover from a surgical procedure include:

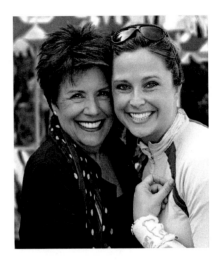

- Be sure you talk to your team before the surgical procedure so you know exactly what to expect after the surgery.
- After lung surgery, the incision area may be sore. A cold pack for 20 minutes at a time may help relieve the swelling at the site. Talk to your surgeon to make sure this is something you can do.
- It may help if you sleep with your head and shoulders raised. This may help your lungs to expand more fully and allow you to breathe better.
- Unless your surgeon says you should stay in bed, be sure to get up in a chair several times a day and walk a little more each day. Unless your condition requires that you stay in bed, you will recover faster if you get up and moving as soon as possible after surgery.
- The first day or two after surgery, you should take pain medicine regularly in order to make it easier to move; however, the sooner you stop taking pain medicine the more energy you will have.

- Eat small meals often. These small meals will allow you to have energy throughout the day without having a full stomach that may interfere with your breathing. As you eat more frequent but smaller meals, be sure you are drinking lots of fluid.
- Keep all appointments with your healthcare team and report any symptoms that you think are not normal following your surgery!

Information presented in *Navigating Lung Cancer 360° of Hope* is not intended as a substitute for the advice given by your health care provider. We recommend you follow the instructions provided to you by your healthcare team. Contact your physician with any questions or concerns.

## CHEMOTHERAPY FOR THE TREATMENT OF NSCLC

Chemotherapy can be used to treat lung cancer stages I - IV NSCLC and SCLC, limited and extensive.

### When is chemotherapy used to treat lung cancer?

Your oncologist may use chemotherapy to destroy or control growth of cancer in the body. Chemotherapy is a cancer treatment that uses drugs in pill form or intravenously (IV inserted into a vein or delivered through a port in the chest wall) to stop the growth of cancer cells, either by killing the cells or by stopping them from dividing. Your oncologist may also refer to chemotherapy as systemic therapy because it circulates throughout the body. If you receive chemotherapy, your oncologist may prescribe only one of these drugs. Most of the time, your oncologist will prescribe chemotherapy drugs in some combination of drugs. When you receive several different chemotherapy drugs, this combination of drugs is called a *chemotherapy regimen*.

Questions for your physician regarding chemotherapy:

- Will I have one drug or a combination of drugs?
- What are the benefits of chemotherapy?
- When will treatment start and how long will it last?
- How often will I receive chemotherapy?
- Where do I go for treatment?
- Will I need someone to help me get home after my chemotherapy?
- How will we know the treatment is working?
- What side effects should I tell you about?
- Can I prevent or treat any of the side effects?
- Will I have side effects after the treatment is completed?
- Can I take vitamins while I am on chemotherapy?
- Do I have to eat certain foods or avoid certain foods?

Your oncologist will determine the dose and schedule of your chemotherapy regimen based on the type, stage and molecular profile of your tumor. Usually, you will receive your chemotherapy treatment in cycles, with each period of treatment followed by a recovery period. You will receive a first chemotherapy regimen called a first-line treatment. If the first-line treatment is not effective, you may receive another combination of chemotherapy drugs called a second-line treatment. The Food and Drug Administration (FDA) classifies different chemotherapy drugs as first- or second-line treatments. This means each chemotherapy drug has been determined to be effective as either a first- or second-line treatment.

In NSCLC, chemotherapy drugs can be used as *neoadjuvant therapy*, which is treatment <u>before</u> surgery. Your oncologist may prescribe neoadjuvant therapy to shrink the tumor so that surgery will be easier or more effective. Neoadjuvant chemotherapy treatments are usually used in stage IIIA cancer. Your doctor will use these drugs before surgery to kill cancer cells in lymph nodes in the chest before surgery. After the chemotherapy, surgery will be done and more chemotherapy will probably be done. Sometimes, your oncologist may also prescribe radiation after the surgery and chemotherapy treatments.

Chemotherapy drugs may be used as *adjuvant therapy*. Adjuvant therapy is any therapy that is started <u>after</u> surgery. Your oncologist may prescribe adjuvant therapy to kill cancer cells that may not have been removed during surgery or which may have spread from the primary tumor.

> *"Numerous clinical trials have shown statistical improvement in outcomes for using at least two drugs (doublets) for adjuvant treatment in stage IB, stage II and stage III disease as well as in first-line treatment for stage IV disease."* —Shane Dormady, MD, PhD

Your surgeon may not be able to remove late stage non-small cell lung cancers by surgery. In this case, your oncologist will probably prescribe chemotherapy to try to destroy cancer cells or control the growth of the tumor. A number of chemotherapy regimens can be used to treat non-small cell lung cancer. These are usually used for stages III - IV for NSCLC. For information on SCLC treatments, see the chapter titled the Small Cell Lung Cancer—Treatments.

If you have a good response after the first-line treatment, your oncologist may prescribe *maintenance therapy*. There are two types of maintenance therapy: continuation maintenance and switch maintenance. *Continuation maintenance therapy* means that your oncologist will continue using at least one of the chemotherapy drugs you received during your first-line treatment. *Switch maintenance* means that your oncologist will prescribe a different chemotherapy drug – one that was not part of your first-line treatment.

### What kinds of chemotherapy might be used to treat me?
Your oncologist may prescribe one or more chemotherapy drugs that you will receive in your vein (IV or intravenous) or by pill. If your treatment involves drugs in the vein, you will receive these drugs in the hospital or in your cancer center's infusion center. If your treatment involves drugs in pill form, you will be able to take these at home.

### What specific FDA-approved drugs, or chemotherapies, are approved for NSCLC?
We understand the following list may be overwhelming. It is important to understand that for NSCLC, a platinum-based chemotherapy is the backbone of the "recipe" and with first-line therapy your doctor will add another drug to the platinum-drug (e.g. Alimta®, Taxol®, or Gemzar®). As you move to second-, third- and fourth-line therapy, some of the drugs are just used one at a time.

| Approved for | Generic Name | Brand Name(s) |
|---|---|---|
| NSCLC | Alectinib | Alecensa® (Approved for patients with *ALK*-rearranged metastatic NSCLC who have progressed on or are intolerant to Crizotinib (Xalkori®) |
| NSCLC | Brigatinib | Alunbrig™ (ALK positive LC patients—after progression on Crizotinib (Xalkori®) |
| NSCLC | Bevacizumab | Avastin® (Targeted therapy used in combination with carboplatin and paclitaxel) |
| Both NSCLC & SCLC | Carboplatin | Paraplat, Paraplatin® |
| NSCLC | Certinib | Zykadia® (Targeted therapy for those with *EML4-ALK* fusion gene) |
| NSCLC | Cetuximab | Erbitux® (Targeted therapy approved for use in other types of cancer but is used in clinical trials for those with NSCLC) |
| Both NSCLC & SCLC | Cisplatin | Platinol®, Platinol A-Q |
| NSCLC | Crizotinib | Xalkori® (Targeted therapy for those with *EML4-ALK* fusion gene and those who are *ROS1*-positive) |
| Both NSCLC & SCLC | Docetaxel | Taxotere® (Approved for use in combination with either cisplatin or carboplatin for NSCLC) |
| NSCLC | Durvalumab | Imfinzi™ (For patients with advanced, unresectable Stage III that had not progressed following standard platinum-based chemotherapy concurrent with radiation therapy) |
| NSCLC | Erlotinib Hydrochloride | Tarceva® (Targeted therapy for those with *EGFR* mutation) |
| Both NSCLC & SCLC | Etoposide | Toposar®, VePesid® |
| NSCLC | Everolimus | Afinitor® (Approved for the treatment of adult patients with progressive, well-dif-ferntiated non-functional, neuroendocrine tumors of gastrointestinal or lung origin with unresectable, locally advanced or metastatic disease) |
| NSCLC | Gefitinib | Iressa™ (Targeted therapy for those with *EGFR* mutation) |

| Approved for | Generic Name | Brand Name(s) |
| --- | --- | --- |
| Both NSCLC & SCLC | Gemcitabine Hydrochloride | Gemzar® (Approved for use in combination with either cisplatin or carboplatin for NSCLC) |
| NSCLC | Gilotrif | Afatinib® (Targeted therapy for those with *EGFR* mutation) |
| Both NSCLC & SCLC | Ifosfamide | Ifex® |
| NSCLC | Irinotecan | Camptosar®, CPT-11 |
| NSCLC | Lorlotinib | ALK positive LC patients—after progression on patients previously treated with one or more ALK inhibitors |
| NSCLC | NAB-Paxlitaxel | Abraxane® (Approved for use in combination with carboplatin) |
| NSCLC | Methotrexate | Abitrexate, Folex®, Folex PFS, Methotrexate LPF, Mexate®, Mexate A-Q |
| NSCLC | Necitumumab | Portrazza™ (Approved for treatment of advanced, metastatic squamous NSCLC patients who have not been previously treated for advanced lung cancer |
| NSCLC | Nivolumab | Opdivo® (First immunotherapy drug targeting lung cancer) |
| NSCLC | Osimertinib | Tagrisso™ (Approved for patients whose disease has progressed on *EGFR*-targeted therapies |
| NSCLC | Pembrolizumab | Keytruda® (Approved for patients with advanced, metastatic NSCLC whose disease has progressed after other treatments (chemotherapy or targeted therapy) and whose tumors express the protein PDL1 |
| NSCLC | Pemetrexed Disodium | Alimta® (Approved for use in combination with either cisplatin or carboplatin for NSCLC) |
| NSCLC | Ramucirumab | Cyramza® (Approved for use in combination with docetaxel for NSCLC) |
| Both NSCLC & SCLC | Topotecan Hydrochloride | Hycamtin® |
| Both NSCLC & SCLC | Vinblastine | Velban™ |
| NSCLC | Vinorelbine | Navelbine® (Approved to be used alone or for use in combination with cisplatin ) |

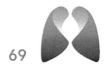

Advantages of chemotherapy treatments:

- May cure the cancer
- Can slow the cancer's growth
- May keep the cancer from spreading
- Can kill cancer cells that may have spread to other parts of the body from the original tumor
- Can shrink the tumor prior to surgery
- Can destroy any cancer cells that are still present after surgery and/or radiation
- Can relieve symptoms caused by the cancer

Disadvantages of chemotherapy treatments:

- May not be effective
- May need more than one chemotherapy regimen
- Side effects of chemotherapy drugs

What to expect with your chemotherapy regimen:

- If your treatment plan consists of many treatments with chemotherapy drugs in your veins, your oncologist may suggest that you have a permanent IV site, or port, put under your skin near your collarbone. This port allows easy access to your blood stream and protects the veins in your arms.
- Unless you develop complications that require that you be in the hospital, your healthcare team will probably give you your IV treatments on an outpatient basis at the hospital or cancer center.
- If your chemotherapy drug is in pill form, your oncologist will tell you how and when to take the pill. You will be able to take the pills at home.

**Possible side effects of chemotherapy:**

Side effects of chemotherapy will depend on the type and length of your treatment and your body's own reaction to the chemotherapy drugs. Although not an exhaustive list, you may experience some of the following:

- Fatigue
- Feeling weak, loss of strength
- Nausea and vomiting
- Hair loss
- Drop in white-blood cells, increasing chance of infection
- Drop in red-blood cells, increasing chance of anemia
- Skin and nail changes
- Peripheral neuropathy (tingling, burning, weakness or numbness in your hands/feet)

**Possible long-term effects of chemotherapy:**

- Menopause
- Infertility
- Damage to your heart or lungs
- Bone disease (brittle/necrotic)

## RADIATION THERAPY FOR THE TREATMENT OF LUNG CANCER

**When is radiation therapy used to treat lung cancer?**

Your oncologist may prescribe traditional radiation therapy as part of your treatment plan. Radiation therapy treats lung cancer by using high-energy x-ray beams to destroy cancerous tumors. Because radiation is focused directly on the tumor, you may hear it referred to as local therapy as opposed to chemotherapy that goes through your whole body and is called a systemic therapy. Cancer experts classify radiation therapy as a local therapy because it is aimed directly at the tumor.

Radiation treatments are sometimes given along with chemotherapy. This is known as combination or combined modality therapy. Combination therapy may have more side

Questions to ask your physician regarding radiation therapies:

- What is the probability that radiation therapy will work for me? If it works, what are the chances that the cancer will come back in the same place or other places?
- What are the chances that the cancer will spread if I do not have radiation therapy?
- How will the radiation therapy be given?
- How many treatments will I receive per week and for how long?
- What side effects should I expect and how do I manage them?
- Will I also need other treatments, such as chemotherapy, surgery, or hormone therapy? If so, when will I receive them and in what order?
- Will I need a special diet during or after my radiation treatment?
- Can I drive myself to and from the treatment facility? Do you recommend I bring a friend or family member?
- Will I be able to continue my normal activities during treatment? If not, how soon after treatment will I be able to resume them such as work, aerobic exercise and sexual activity?
- How can I expect to feel during treatment and in the weeks following radiation therapy?
- What symptoms/problems after radiation should I tell you about?
- After my treatment is completed, how often will I need to return for checkups?

effects than radiation or chemotherapy alone, but can be more effective at destroying the cancer cells.

## Are there different types of radiation?

## External Beam Radiation

The most common kind of radiation treatment to treat lung cancer is "external beam radiation." This treatment uses a machine called a linear accelerator to treat your lung cancer with high-energy photons, or "x-rays." The high-energy x-rays are aimed at the tumor and destroy the DNA of the cancer cells. External beam radiation can be used to treat both small cell and non-small cell lung cancers of all stages.

Your radiation oncologist will talk to you about the type of treatment that is recommended in your particular case. Your external beam radiation treatment will usually last for 6 to 8 weeks. Types of external beam radiation include:

- **3-D Conformal Radiation Therapy**
  One of the most common types of external beam radiation therapy is three-dimensional conformal radiotherapy (3DCRT). This type of radiation therapy is a complicated treatment process that begins with x-rays that your radiation oncologist will use to create 3-D images of the tumor and the normal tissues around it. Your healthcare team will use these 3-D pictures to plan your individual treatment that will deliver radiation directly to your tumor and the area at risk around it. With 3DCRT, your radiation oncologist will be able to use multiple beams to deliver radiation to the tumor while limiting the amount of radiation to the healthy tissue around it.

- **Intensity-Modulated Radiation Therapy (IMRT)**
  Intensity-modulated radiation therapy, most commonly called IMRT, is an advanced form of 3DCRT. Your radiation oncologist will use specialized software and hardware to focus small "beamlets" of radiation to treat only the tumor while limiting dose to the healthy tissue around the tumor. This allows your doctor to treat tumors that might have been untreatable in the past because they were too close to healthy organs.

- In some cases, there may be fewer side effects than with conventional radiation treatments. Treatment times for each IMRT treatment may be longer than with other techniques because daily set-up is very precise and requires multiple measurements.

73

- **Image Guidance Radiation Therapy (IGRT)**

  One of the problems with treating lung cancer with radiation treatment is that the tumor moves as you breathe. With Image Guidance Radiation Therapy (IGRT) tracking, the radiation beam turns on <u>only</u> when the tumor is in the path of the beam. IGRT is another radiation treatment that targets the tumor only, limiting the exposure of normal tissue around the tumor.

- **Volumetric Arc Therapy (VMAT)**

  Volumetric Arc Therapy (VMAT) is the most advanced form of IMRT. It allows for treatment of the tumor as the radiation machine is moving. This means your treatment may be faster.

## Radiosurgery

Another way to treat lung cancer is with radiosurgery, also called "stereotactic radiotherapy." Radiosurgery does not involve actual surgery with a knife, but instead uses many pinpoint radiation beams that focus on one small area and treat it with a very high dose of radiation.

When radiosurgery is used for cancers in the lung or elsewhere in the body (outside of the head), it is called "stereotactic body radiation therapy" or SBRT. SBRT can be given with a traditional radiation device or with a machine especially designed for radiosurgery. SBRT can be used in place of traditional surgery in some patients with early stage disease who either cannot or choose not to have surgery. New studies released in 2011 showed that radiosurgery has results that are as good as or better than traditional surgery in some stage I patients.[12,13]

A typical radiosurgery course of treatment takes 1 to 5 treatments, as opposed to 6 or 7 weeks with other types of external beam radiation. Each SBRT treatment may last several hours.

## What to expect with Radiation Therapy

External beam radiation is usually given once per day, Monday through Friday, for 6 to 8 weeks. During treatment, you will be lying on a table and the machine will move around you. You will hear some noises from the machine, but the treatment itself is painless, much like having a chest x-ray or dental x-ray. In order to make sure you are in the proper position, your radiology technician may place small dots in the form of a tattoo in order to aim the radiation beam at exactly the same spot each time you receive radiation therapy. You will be asked to lie still for 15 to 30 minutes depending on the length of the treatment. Although each individual treatment is painless, a small dose of radiation is given each day and you should be aware of the possible side effects that may develop during the course of your treatment:

- Your skin may look and feel as if it has been sunburned. You will be given skin creams and instructions on how to manage this, and it will go away within in a few weeks after your treatment is complete.
- Mild or moderate fatigue may begin after the first few weeks of treatment. This fatigue will peak by the end of treatment. Approximately 4 to 8 weeks following the end of treatment, your fatigue should be much better. Fatigue may be worse if you are receiving a combination of chemotherapy and radiation.
- Your esophagus is often exposed to radiation during lung cancer treatment.
- This exposure to the radiation can result in temporary sore throat and pain with
- swallowing that you may first notice 3 to 4 weeks into your treatment. You may
- find that soft foods or liquids are easier to swallow during this time, and your
- doctor may prescribe medication to help with discomfort. Your sore throat
- and difficulty swallowing should be better within 2 to 3 weeks after your treatments are completed.
- You may develop a temporary cough or change in breathing during radiation. This is usually managed with cough medications and sometimes a short course of steroids.
- Radiation pneumonitis is a radiation pneumonia

caused by treatment. This complication occurs in 5 to 15% of patients and typically happens 2 to 6 months <u>after</u> your treatment is complete.[14] This is a particularly important side effect because, if it is not treated, pneumonitis can be very serious. If you develop shortness of breath, chest pain when you breathe, cough or a low-grade fever after finishing radiation, be sure to report the symptoms to your oncologist. Pneumonitis is usually diagnosed with a chest x-ray and it is treated with steroids. With appropriate treatment, you will probably not have any lasting problems.

> Ask your oncologist to check you for radiation pneumonitis during your 6 month appointment after radiation treatment.

- Radiation fibrosis is scarring of the lung that develops after radiation treatment. The amount of scarring depends on how much of your normal lung had to be treated, and the dose of radiation to that lung. Depending on the severity of the fibrosis, it can cause shortness of breath and coughing. Your oncologist may want you to be on oxygen if scarring develops.

## Advantages of Radiation Therapy

- May cure the cancer
- May be used to shrink tumors to relieve pain or make surgery possible
- May be used as a targeted therapy to decrease the amount of time needed to give radiation, and leave healthy tissue unharmed.

## Disadvantages of Radiation Therapy

- Side effects such asthose listed above
- Unless you receive radiosurgery, you may spend time at appointments every day for several weeks

## Brain metastases

Radiation therapy is commonly used to treat brain metastases from lung cancer. In some cases, radiation is used to try to prevent brain metastases in people who are at high risk for developing them.

**External beam radiation** is used for treatment of the entire brain. Standard whole brain radiation is used for tumors that can be seen as well as for abnormal cells that can only be seen through a microscope. Your radiation oncologist will prescribe treatments lasting 2 to 4 weeks. Whole brain radiation may result in memory and cognition deficits unless hippocampal avoidance whole brain radiation is used instead of standard whole brain radiation. Avoiding radiation dose to the hippocampus minimizes memory and cognition deficits.

**Radiosurgery** is focused treatment that targets only the visible tumors. Typically, tumors up to 3 to 4 cm can be treated. There are various ways to treat brain metastases with commercially available radiosurgery devices including linear accelerator-based treatment, Gamma Knife®,Cyberknife®, Novalis and TrueBeam™. All of these treatments use pinpoint x-ray beams to target tumors with a high dose of radiation, and there are no clinical outcome data favoring one over another.

At times, radiosurgery is used in combination with whole brain radiation therapy for brain metastases. This combination can work well because whole brain radiation therapy treats the microscopic disease with a low dose of radiation and radiosurgery can deliver a high dose directly to the visible tumors.

Side effects from radiation to the brain vary depending on the type of treatment, but can include fatigue, weakness, hair loss, and neurologic effects including memory loss and speech problems.

> It is very important to understand your treatment options for brain metastasis.
>
> Ask your doctor which treatment regime is available to you and best for your situation.

**New and experimental types of radiation treatment for lung cancer**

### Brachytherapy

Brachytherapy is the delivery of radiation treatment using radioactive seeds. These seeds may be placed in the target area and left for a specific length of time or may be left in the area permanently. Unlike external beam radiation, brachytherapy delivers radiation from inside the body.

### Endoluminal high dose rate (HDR) brachytherapy

In HDR brachytherapy treatment, your pulmonologist places a high dose radioactive seed into the lung tumor using a small catheter through a bronchoscope. The seed is left in temporarily and then removed.

### Mesh brachytherapy

This type of brachytherapy uses permanent radiation seeds (called a mesh) that are placed on the area where the tumor had been after a lung cancer is removed surgically. Mesh brachytherapy delivers a precise dose of radiation and reduces the risk of recurrence.

### NanoKnife Electroporation

The NanoKnife® Irreversible Electroporation (IRE) System is a treatment that uses electrical energy to destroy soft tissue tumors. Probes are placed in the tumor and then brief electrical pulses are sent through the probes.

## PULMONARY THERAPY

Interventional pulmonology is a specialty within pulmonary medicine that focuses on treating lung cancer and other airway diseases performed by a pulmonary medicine doctor who has additional advanced training in minimally invasive techniques and will be involved with your team in diagnosis, staging and treatment of lung cancer. A pulmonologist will usually do any number of procedures that will assist your oncologist, thoracic surgeon or radiation oncologist from biopsy procedures to treatment or symptom management.

The advantages of interventional pulmonary therapy are (1) less invasive procedure, (2) more precise biopsies and delivery of treatment, and (3) decreased recovery time. Your pulmonologist will describe the benefits and risks of each procedure.

### Biopsy Procedures

**Electromagnetic Navigation Bronchoscopy™ Procedure**: Also known as ENB™ procedures, Electromagnetic Navigation Bronchoscopy™ procedures are performed by a pulmonologist or thoracic surgeon. ENB™ procedures provide a minimally invasive approach to accessing difficult-to-reach areas of the lung aiding in the diagnosis of lung disease.

Covidien's LungGPS™ technology used in the superDimension™ navigation system is state-of-the-art, and proven. Ask your doctor if an ENB™ procedure is appropriate for you. Visit the Our Generous Supporters chapter of this guidebook for more information on Covidien's technology.

Using your CAT scan, Covidien's superDimension™ navigation system with LungGPS™ technology creates a roadmap of your lungs, like a GPS (Global Positioning System) does in a car. That roadmap guides your physician through the airways of your lungs to the nodule. Your physician will insert a bronchoscope through your mouth or nose and into your lungs. With the bronchoscope in place, your physician is able to navigate through your natural airways to the lung nodule. Using tiny instruments, your physician will take a sample of the nodule for testing. In some cases, small markers may be placed near the lung nodule to help guide a physician delivering follow-up treatment or therapy.

Unlike a traditional bronchoscopy, the devices used in an ENB procedure create a real-time, image-guided map for doctors to access the deepest regions of your lungs. This allows them to see tumors and nodes that can't be seen or accessed by a traditional bronchoscope; making the need for more invasive techniques and exploratory surgeries unnecessary. This technology may be suitable for you if:

- You cannot undergo more aggressive procedures
- You have multiple tumors
- You want a diagnosis and/or staging before undergoing surgery
- You may be a candidate for stereotactic radiosurgery for fiducial marker placement at the time of biopsy
- You want to obtain additional lung tissue for genetic testing

**Endobronchial Ultrasound (EBUS) and Radial Probe Ultrasound (REBUS)**
With EBUS or REBUS, your pulmonologist uses a special ultrasound equipped bronchoscope. Your doctor may use this technique to do biopsies on multiple lesions. The procedure is much more accurate and the risk of puncturing a blood vessel is minimal, because the pulmonologist can see the needle as it is placed inside the tumor. Your doctor may use this technique to biopsy lymph nodes in the middle of the chest (EBUS) or in peripheral lung areas (REBUS).

### Narrow band imaging

Narrow band imaging uses a specialized light at specific wavelengths that can detect abnormal blood vessels in the airway. These abnormal vessels may indicate tumor growth. Using these abnormal vessels, the pulmonologist may be able to guide a biopsy during bronchoscopy. Although not fully validated by scientific data, this technique may be used as a supplemental tool in some programs.

## Treatment & Symptom Management Procedures

### Argon Plasma Coagulation (APC)

For an APC procedure, your pulmonologist will use this technology to destroy tumors or stop bleeding. Using APC, your pulmonologist will use an argon gas jet to apply heat to specific areas without having to make direct contact with the area.

As a result, the pulmonologist can treat a larger area,which will often shorten the procedure time.

### Cryosurgery, laser

Using a bronchoscope, your pulmonologist may use cryotherapy to destroy tumors in your airways by freezing the tissue. The pulmonologist will apply a super-cooled probe over the entire surface of the tumor. This procedure is often used with argon plasma coagulation to open any airways that are blocked by a tumor or by scar tissue that forms as part of the healing process.

## Fiducial placement for Stereotactic Body Radiation (SBRT)

Some tumors cannot be treated through traditional surgery, but may respond very well to stereotactic radiosurgery. To make sure that SBRT is delivered to the exact location of the tumor, Covidien's SuperLock™ fiducial markers are placed in or near the tumor and can be placed at the same time as your ENB™ procedure for biopsy using Covidien's superDimension™ system. A fiducial marker is simply a small gold seed or platinum coil that is placed around a tumor to act as a radiologic landmark.

> Covidien's LungGPS™ technology used in the superDimension™ navigation system is state-of-the-art, and proven. Ask your doctor if an ENB™ procedure for the placement of markers is appropriate for you. Visit the Our Generous Supporters chapter of this guidebook for more information on Covidien's technology.

## High dose rate (HDR) brachytherapy, also called Image-Guided Brachytherapy (IGBT)

Using some sort of radiology tool or x-ray, your pulmonologist will place a catheter into the lung tumor and deliver high dose radiation by passing radioactive seeds through the catheter. This technique minimizes damage to lung tissue and delivers higher dose of radiation to the tumor; as a result, more cancer cells are destroyed.

## Airway Stenting

Airway stents are small, expandable tubes that your pulmonologist may use to open bronchial tubes (airways) that are occluded or narrowed due to the lung tumor or scar tissue. Some covered stents can also be used to prevent the cancer from growing back into the breathing tube and compromising lung function.

### Pleuroscopy

When a laparoscopy is performed in the chest, it is called pleuroscopy or medical thoracoscopy. A small instrument with a camera is inserted into the chest cavity through a very small incision, enabling the pulmonologist to perform diagnostic and therapeutic procedures inside the chest.

### Balloon bronchoplasty

A balloon bronchoplasty is a technique that your pulmonologist may use to open a narrow airway using a balloon. It is very similar to how coronary arteries are opened during a heart angioplasty. Bronchoplasty is particularly useful when an airway is narrowed because of scarring after a tracheotomy, for example. Depending on the location of the narrowing, the dilation (or widening) of the airway can be performed using a flexible or rigid bronchoscope. It can also be done prior to stent placement.

## OTHER TREATMENT OPTIONS

### Photodynamic therapy (PDT)

Photodynamic therapy is a cancer treatment that uses a drug called a photosensitizer or porfimer sodium (brand name Photofrin®) and a certain type of light to kill cancer cells. After it is injected into a vein, the photosensitizer drug is exposed to certain wavelengths of light and becomes active. This activation of the photosensitizer produces a certain kind of oxygen that kills the tumor and nearby cells or blood vessels that are feeding the tumor. The photosensitizer may also activate your immune system to destroy the tumor cells.

PDT is usually only used on small tumors since the light that is used cannot pass through bigger tumors. Your doctor may use PDT to relieve the symptoms of a non-small lung cancer that is blocking your airway. To do this, the doctor will use a bronchoscope to shine the light on the tumor. Your doctor may use Photodynamic therapy along with other therapies like chemotherapy and/or radiation.

83

PDT is performed at only select academic centers in the United States. Generally, a pulmonologist or interventional radiologist performs the procedure though, occasionally, a surgeon will be certified to do so.

The Food and Drug Administration (FDA) has approved PDT for the treatment of non-small cell lung cancer when the tumor cannot be treated using other treatment options. The FDA also approved PDT to relieve symptoms caused by these tumors when they block airways in the lung.

Advantages of PDT:

- Causes little damage to healthy tissue
- Is less invasive than surgery to remove tumors
- Can be done on an outpatient basis
- Provides targeted therapy directly to the tumor

Disadvantages of PDT:

- Cannot treat very large tumors or tumors in body cavities because the light
- used in PDT can only pass through a small amount of tissue
- Generally, PDT cannot be used for tumors that have metastasized or spread
- to other areas

## What to expect with PDT:

- PDT is usually performed during an outpatient visit or short hospital stay
- A member of your healthcare team will inject the photosensitizer drug 24 to 72 hours before the procedure
- The drug will be absorbed by all cells but stays in cancer cells longer than normal cells
- After the photosensitizer has left most of the normal cells, the tumor is exposed to the special light to activate the drug and kill the tumor cells

## Side effects of PDT:

- Porfimer sodium may make your skin and eyes sensitive to light for about 6 weeks after injection. You should avoid direct sunlight during the time of your treatments.
- The treatment may cause burns, swelling, pain, and scarring in otherwise healthy tissue.
- PDT may cause temporary side effects, including coughing, trouble swallowing, stomach pain, painful breathing, or shortness of breath.

To learn more about Photodynamic therapy for cancer visit the National Cancer Institute website at http://www.cancer.gov/cancertopics/factsheet/Therapy/photodynamic.

## Vaccine therapy

Research and clinical trials are being conducted in the United States on the use of a "lung cancer vaccine." In this treatment, the vaccine is used to stimulate antibody production. The antibodies produced by your immune system target the cancer cells and destroy them. See the Clinical Trials chapter for more information on how to find clinical trials in your area.

## SUMMARY OF TREATMENT OPTIONS FOR NSCLC: STAGES I, II, III, AND IV

The following is a summary of treatment options for individuals diagnosed with NSCLC.

**Stage 0:** Stage 0 lung cancer is lung cancer found only in the lining of your air passages. Most lung cancer is diagnosed at later stages; stage 0 lung cancer patients are usually discovered through sputum cytology. If you are diagnosed with stage 0 lung cancer, it is probably because you participated in a lung screening trial or because you are considered to be at high risk. Stage 0 lung cancer is also known as carcinoma in situ.

*Carcinoma in situ* are tumors that are present in only a few layers of cells. These tumors have not grown (or metastasized) outside the lining of your air passages however, they may progress to invasive cancer. Standard treatments may include surgical resection usually by segmentectomy or wedge resection. The goal of the treatment is to remove as little normal tissue as possible. Occasionally, if the tumor is more centrally located, your surgeon may have to do a lobectomy.

**Stage I:** If you are diagnosed with stage I lung cancer, this means that the cancer is located in one lung and has not spread to your lymph nodes or outside of the chest. At this early stage, surgery is usually the treatment of choice. Be aware that your oncologist may recommend a multi-treatment approach in which two or more types of treatment are combined. Your team will discuss with you the type of surgery they recommend and whether the addition of chemotherapy or radiation is appropriate. Talk to your oncologist about the potential risks and benefits for each treatment option.

Surgical removal of the cancer may be accomplished through various techniques including segmentectomy (removal of a small segment of the lung), lobectomy (removal of a lobe of the lung) or pneumonectomy (removal of the entire lung). When determining treatment, your oncologist will take into account your age and general health, as well as where the cancer is located. Your oncologist and surgeon will try to remove as little of the lung as possible in order to preserve as much lung function as possible. Your oncologist will be able to tell you if you are not a surgical candidate based on your age or on concurrent health conditions that might make surgery too risky. If you are not a good candidate for surgery, your oncologist will talk to you about using newer imaging techniques such as positron emission tomography (PET) scan that can more accurately stage your cancer so that radiation can be used.

The five-year survival rate for stage I NSCLC is approximately 60 to 80% with surgery.[15] However, even in early stages of lung cancer, cancer cells may have spread outside the lung and may not be found. Therefore, your oncologist may recommend chemotherapy before or after surgery.

**Stage II:** About 30% of lung cancer are diagnosed at this stage.[16]

Stage II tumor is one that has been found in one lung and may be present in lymph nodes on the same side of the chest but not in the lymph nodes of the mediastinum. Your oncologist will probably identify surgery as the best first-line treatment if your age and general health are good. However, if you are diagnosed with stage II NSCLC, you may require more than one treatment type to increase the effectiveness of treatment and prevent recurrence.

Surgical options are usually the same for stage II as stage I. Surgery is the treatment of choice for patients with stage II NSCLC. A lobectomy, pneumonectomy, or segmental resection, wedge resection, or sleeve resection may be performed as appropriate. Your oncologist will do a careful assessment of your overall health to determine the risks and benefits of surgery. For stage II NSCLC tumors, surgical removal results in 20 to 30% of patients being alive without return of the cancer within 5 years of surgery.[16]

If it is determined that surgery may not have removed all cancer cells, your oncologist may recommend chemotherapy and/or radiation as further treatment. If your oncologist determines that you are not a good candidate for surgery, he may recommend stereotactic body radiation therapy (SBRT) to kill any remaining cancer cells.

**Stage III:** About 30% of lung cancer is diagnosed at stage IIIA or IIIB.[17]

**Stage IIIA:** A stage IIIA tumor has extended into lymph nodes in the tracheal area outside the lung. These lymph nodes may be around the diaphragm or chest wall and will be on the same side of the body on which the cancer started. Some stage IIIA NSCLC tumors can be treated with surgery and others cannot.

If the stage IIIA tumor can be treated with surgery, your oncologist may recommend some combination of surgery, chemotherapy, radiation or a clinical trial of new treatments. Because all tumors are different, your oncologist and treatment team will decide what treatments should be done and in what order they will be most effective.

If the stage IIIA tumor cannot be treated with surgery, your oncologist may recommend some combination of chemotherapy, external radiation, internal radiation or a clinical trial of new treatments. Because all tumors are different, your oncologist and treatment team will decide what treatments should be done and in what order they will be most effective.

**Stage IIIB:** A stage IIIB tumor is a cancer that has extended into lymph nodes in the neck or in the opposite lung from where the cancer started. It is very common for your oncologist to provide more than one type of treatment if your tumor is a stage IIIB NSCLC. Some combination of chemotherapy, internal or external radiation, surgery or clinical trials may be prescribed as part of your treatment plan. Timing of each treatment will be based on your age and general health.

**Stage IV:** About 40% of NSCLC is diagnosed at stage IV.[18]

If you are diagnosed with a stage IV NSCLC tumor, the cancer has spread into both lungs or more distant parts of the body. A diagnosis of a stage IV tumor must include one or more of the following:

- There is at least one tumor in each lung;
- Cancer cells are found in fluid around the lungs or the heart;
- Cancer has spread to other parts of the body.

Again, your individual treatment plan will be developed based on your age and general health. Treatment options for stage IV NSCLC may include radiation therapy, chemotherapy, and targeted therapy. Radiation therapy is used mainly for pain control rather than an intent to cure. Treatment options may include combinations of chemotherapy, *EGFR* inhibitors if you have an *EGFR* mutation (see Molecular Testing section), external beam radiation therapy for local tumor growth (see Radiation Therapy section), or brachytherapy if you have tumors that obstruct your airway (see Radiation Therapy section). New drugs and combinations of treatments are being studied and a clinical trial may be available to you.

**Stage IV disease complications**

**Bone metastases**

### Palliative radiation

Often stage IV patients have tumors in their bones, or bone metastases. Many times these bone metastases result in pain, decreased ability to move, anemia, bone fractures and in some cases, if near the spine, paralysis. Treatment for these tumors is usually radiation therapy for several days to relieve pain and shrink the tumor. Chemotherapy can also shrink bone metastases.

## Brittle bones

Chemotherapy and complications from lung cancer can lead to brittle bones, or osteoporosis. Your oncologist may prescribe one of a number of drugs to decrease your chance of developing brittle bones. Ask your oncologist if one of these medicines might be right for you.

> Monthly infusions of zoledronic acid (Zometa®) or subcutaneous injections of denosumab (Xgeva®) are used in patients with bone metastases to prevent new bone lesions from forming and to help heal existing bone lesions.

*Note:* Before taking one of these medicines, your oncologist may recommend supplements to improve your levels of calcium and vitamin D. Talk to your oncologist about having dental work done before starting any of the medications for brittle bones since the drugs normally given may cause breakdown of the jaw bone resulting in loose teeth, swelling and infection of the jaw and gums, and loss of gum tissue. Be sure your dentist knows that you are taking (or will be taking) one of the drugs for brittle bones.

## Wasting syndrome, or *cachexia*

Wasting syndrome is the loss of body mass that cannot be reversed by eating correctly. This syndrome may cause weight loss, muscle wasting, also known as atrophy, extreme fatigue and weakness, and loss of appetite. If you develop wasting syndrome, you may not be able to tolerate treatments as well so it is important that your team treat this syndrome aggressively. If you develop wasting syndrome, your oncologist may prescribe steroids. A few drugs in clinical development and available via clinical trials may prevent wasting syndrome when given with first-line chemotherapy. Ask your physician if participating in a clinical trial for wasting syndrome might be right for you.

## Need for oxygen

For many different reasons, a lung cancer patient may experience the need for oxygen: flying, traveling to a high altitude location, symptoms from fluid build-up in the lung, removal of the lobe of a lung or the entire lung itself or other complications. You may have your physician order an oxygen tank for your use at home and when you travel.

## Pneumonia

Lung cancer can, for many reasons, weaken your immune system, putting you at risk for pneumonia. Pneumonia is an infection of the lung. It is important to go to your doctor to be checked for pneumonia if you experience a continuing or worsening cough, chest pain, difficulty breathing or fever. You may be required to stay in the hospital to receive intravenous (in the vein) antibiotics, or you may be able to be treated at home with oral antibiotics. Pneumonia needs to be treated to avoid more serious issues with breathing and circulatory problems.

## Fluid in or around the lungs, or pleural effusion

This fluid build-up often contains cancer cells. It causes coughing and can cause severe shortness of breath. It may require a surgical procedure, called *pleurodesis*, to essentially 'glue' the lung to its lining to keep fluid build-up from happening. This procedure involves inserting a chest tube to insert chemicals to induce a scar, thus 'gluing' the lung to its lining. The chest tube must remain in for a few days at least until the fluid has completely drained out of the lung. Another option is to have a drainage catheter (tube) inserted into the lung for about 30 days. Each day the patient or a caregiver connects the catheter to a simple vacuum tube that drains the collecting fluid. When not in use there is a cap placed on the tube. This is a good option for patients with pleural effusions to be at home and to continue receiving chemotherapy, if indicated.

### Embolism

Cancer can make your blood thicker than usual and this can lead to blood clots. When a blood clot travels through the blood stream into your lung, it is called a pulmonary embolism. This is similar to a blood clot that becomes lodged in your leg resulting in a deep vein thrombosis.

Symptoms of a pulmonary embolus include sudden shortness of breath, chest pain and coughing up blood. Symptoms of deep vein thrombosis include swelling or severe pain in your leg. Both of these conditions can be treated once they are identified, so if you experience any of these symptoms, you should contact your oncologist <u>immediately</u> so that you can be evaluated and treatment can be started.

## PROTON THERAPY

Proton therapy (also called proton beam therapy) is a type of radiation treatment that uses protons rather than x-rays to treat cancer. A proton is a positively charged particle that is part of an atom, the basic unit of all chemical elements, such as hydrogen or oxygen. At high energy, protons can destroy cancer cells.

Like standard x-ray radiation, proton therapy is a type of external-beam radiation therapy. It painlessly delivers radiation through the skin from a machine outside the body. Protons, however, can target the tumor with lower radiation doses to surrounding normal tissues—approximately 60% lower, depending on the location of the tumor.

Traditional radiation treatment can damage the tissue around the tumor. However, with proton therapy, the protons' energy hits the tumor site, delivering a smaller dose to surrounding healthy tissue. With standard treatment, doctors may need to reduce the radiation dose to limit side effects, resulting from damage to healthy tissue. With treatment using protons, on the other hand, doctors can select an appropriate dose, knowing that there will likely be fewer early and late side effects of radiation on the healthy tissue.

Compared with standard radiation treatment, proton therapy has several benefits. It reduces the risk of radiation damage to healthy tissues; may allow a higher radiation dose to be directed at some types of tumors, which may keep the tumor from growing or spreading; and may result in fewer and less severe side effects (such as low blood counts, fatigue, and nausea) during and after treatment.

(Source: Cancer.net)

*When you are diagnosed with cancer, the most important thing that you can arm yourself with is knowledge and education. The Bonnie J Addario Lung Cancer Foundation provides the tools to arm yourself, through the Patient Education Hand, the website, in person support from staff. The foundation has been a game changer for me.*

*—Jim Brown, survivor*

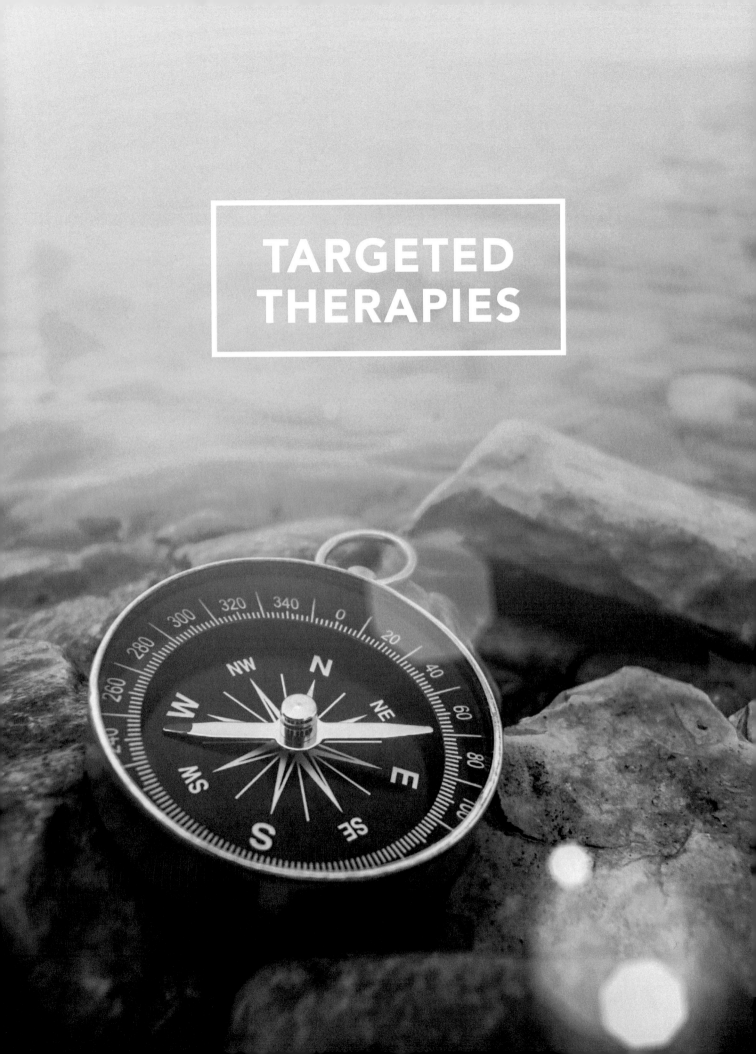

**TARGETED THERAPIES**

*I was diagnosed at Stage IV when I was 28-years old in 2012. I am now NED (No Evidence of Disease). This Foundation was integral in the success of my cancer journey, and I am so grateful to them. During treatment, I promised myself that I would beat this, and then get to work helping patients the way the Foundation had helped me. I was also able to look beyond illness to my dream raising a family. I am now the mother of two baby girls.*

*—Emily Bennett Taylor, survivor*

# TARGETED THERAPIES

## Targeted chemotherapy and personalized medicine

Your oncologist may prescribe "targeted chemotherapy" if your lung cancer is diagnosed as stages III or IV NSCLC. You may also receive these therapies after surgery as maintenance therapy.

## What are targeted therapies?

Targeted therapy is a term you might hear that describes a type of lung cancer treatment that uses drugs to identify and attack cancer cells specifically, while sparing normal cells. Cancer cells can create "mutant proteins" and other genomic abnormalities, such as fusions that cause two unrelated genes to 'fuse'. These mutant proteins and fused genes are what cause cancer cells to grow, divide and spread, and are therefore good targets for drugs that act like "guided missiles" to attack only these "mutant" or abnormal proteins and genes. Although targeted therapies have side effects, they are generally better tolerated than chemotherapy.

> Ask your oncologist to conduct molecular testing to determine if one of the targeted therapies may be right for you.

## Why are targeted therapies important?

Because the genomic alterations driving a cancer, such as protein mutations and gene fusions, in each tumor are different, the treatments for each tumor will be different. These personalized treatments recognize that what works for one type of lung cancer may not work for another. Targeted therapies are a relatively new line of research and treatment for lung cancer. If your oncologist is not familiar with molecular testing and targeted therapies, it is acceptable and advisable to get a second opinion about your treatment options.

## What targeted therapies are available?

Although many gene mutations have been identified in lung cancer tumors, many of the mutations do not have effective targeted therapies identified yet (research is ongoing to find treatments for all of these genomic alterations, with many promising new experimental drugs in clinical trials). Currently, four known mutations have effective targeted therapies available, and approved by the U.S. Food and Drug Administration (FDA). These alterations are *EGFR* mutations, *EGFR* T790M, *ALK* fusions, and *ROS1* fusions. If your tumor tests positive for alterations outside of these four, ask your doctor for clinical trials as a treatment option.

- **Epidermal Growth Factor Receptor (*EGFR*):** About 15 % of patients diagnosed with non-small cell lung cancer have mutations in the *EGFR* gene. Molecular testing for alteration in *EGFR* may tell whether certain types of targeted drugs inhibitors (TKIs) would be beneficial in treating your lung cancer.

If your tumor is *EGFR* mutation negative or "wildtype" (that is, an *EGFR* mutation is not found in the tumor), your oncologist may still prescribe a TKI since the drug may slow cancer growth. Typically, in the case of *EGFR* mutation negative tumors, TKI's will be used as a second-line treatment after chemotherapy.

A blood test, also called a liquid biopsy test, called VeriStrat® is available for advanced non-small cell lung cancer patients. The test looks at protein patterns in the blood and predicts if patients are likely to respond after receiving Tarceva® therapy.

This test is useful for patients in the following groups: *EGFR* wild-type or *EGFR* status unknown, not eligible for chemotherapy, no tumor tissue available, and those with squamous cell.

Because it is a blood test, VeriStrat does not require a tissue biopsy and results are returned in less than 72 hours.

Visit the Our Generous Supporters chapter of this guidebook for more information.
**www.veristratsupport.com**

In June 2016, the U.S. FDA approved a blood/plasma test called Cobas *EGFR* Mutation Test v2 that tests for the presence of specific alterations in the *EGFR* gene (such as exon 19 deletions or exon 21 (L858R) substitution mutations), to identify non-small cell lung cancer (NSCLC) patients eligible for treatment with erlotinib (Tarceva). This blood test or "liquid biopsy" test initially screens patients with metastatic NSCLC for *EGFR* mutations without the need for an invasive biopsy, and is the first ever "liquid biopsy" test approved for use by the FDA. This new test may benefit patients who may be too ill or are otherwise unable to provide a tumor biopsy specimen for *EGFR* testing. If your Cobas *EGFR* liquid biopsy test shows negative results for *EGFR* alterations, you should then have your cancer's *EGFR* status determined from a routine tissue biopsy.

- *EGFR* **T790M:** T790M is a point mutation in the *EGFR* gene that is associated with resistance to epidermal growth factor receptor (*EGFR*)-directed targeted therapies such as erlotinib. If you have an *EGFR* positive lung cancer and have become resistant to the drugs that target the *EGFR* mutation, you may have the T790M "resistance" mutation. Approximately 60% of all patients that stop responding to *EGFR*-directed targeted therapies over time, become resistant to therapies like erlotinib because their cancers have evolved the T790M mutation to bypass treatment and continue to grow. Both tissue and blood tests have been approved as diagnostic tests to look for *EGFR* T790M. If you test positive for *EGFR* T790M, a drug called Tagrisso™ (osimertinib) has been approved to target this mutation.

- *ROS1* **rearrangements:** About 1% to 2% of individuals with non-small cell lung cancer have an abnormality in which the *ROS1* gene is fused to part of another gene These are called, "*ROS1* translocations" or "*ROS1* fusions." The *ROS1* gene makes a protein called ROS, which is found within the membrane of human cells. In March 2016 a targeted therapy called crizotinib or Xalkori was approved for treating *ROS1*-fusion positive lung cancer. If your lung tumors are driven by *ROS1* fusions, check out the Addario Lung Cancer Foundation's Global *ROS1* Initiative at lungcancerfoundation.org/*ROS1* to connect with fellow *ROS1*ers from all over the world, and learn more about other treatment options, clinical trials, and our research study focused on understanding the biology of *ROS1* to identify new treatments for patients like you.

- **Anaplastic Lymphoma Kinase (*ALK*):** About 5% of non-small cell lung cancers are driven by fusions of the *ALK* gene. The *ALK* fusion or re-arrangements produce an abnormal *ALK* protein that causes the cells to spread and grow. Targeted drug therapies have been approved in treating *ALK* positive lung cancer, such as crizotinib (Xalkori) which is a pill that you take twice a day with mild side effects.

Unfortunately, as is the case for most targeted therapies, cancers identify ways to continue to grow despite the targeted treatment. This is called treatment resistance, when *ALK* positive cancers stop responding to treatments like crizotinib. Most *ALK*+ lung cancer patients develop brain metastases upon the development of treatment resistance. The good news is that there are now two new treatments approved for patients whose disease has progressed on crizotinib. These agents- alectinib (Alecensa) and ceritinib (Zykadia) are both oral pills, and are effective treatments for brain metastases as well.

A great deal of research is being done about mutations of proteins and genes that might cause lung cancer.

The following list was created by ALCF with assistance from our contributing authors.

| Abbreviation | Name | Role |
| --- | --- | --- |
| AKT1 | Protein Kinase B | AKT regulates cellular survival and metabolism |
| BRAF | Proto-oncogene B-Raf | A gene that makes a protein called B-Raf. The B-Raf protein helps to send signals inside the cells. These cells are involved in directing the cells growth. |
| CEA | Carcinoembryonic antigen | A blood test used as a tumor marker although not considered reliable enough for diagnosing cancer. |
| c-MET amplified, or c-MET exon 14 skipping | MET or MNNG HOS Transforming gene | MET pathways create new blood vessels that supply nutrients to a tumor and with cell dissociation that may lead to tumor metastasis. The MET pathways are very important in tumor development. |
| ERCC1 | Excision repair cross complementation group 1 | Critical protein in the DNA repair pathway |
| ERCC1 + RRM1 | Excision repair cross complementation group 1 and Ribonucleotidereductase M1 | Both markers are currently being studied to determine their benefit as predictive of benefit from adjuvant treatment in early stage (I-III). |
| HER2 amplified + EGFR | Human Epidermal Growth Factor Receptor 2 + Epidermal Growth Factor Receptor | The measurement of EGFR and HER2 protein expression may have a prognostic value in NSCLC. The two may also have predictive value for identifying patients likely to benefit from an EGFR TKI. |
| NRAS | One of several RAS genes first isolated from human neuroblastoma | The role of NRAS mutations for assistance in selecting or prioritizing cancer treatment, is unknown at this time. |
| PIK3CA, AKT, PTEN | Phosphatidyl 3-kinases (PI3K) | Involved in cell growth and survival. Ask your doctor about the LungMAP clinical trial. |

| Abbreviation | Name | Role |
|---|---|---|
| ROS1 | C-ros oncogene 1, receptor tyrosine kinase | May function as a growth or differentiation factor receptor. |
| RRM1 | Ribonucleotidereductase M1 | Key protein in producing deoxyribonucleotides - the building blocks for DNA. |
| TCF21 | Transcription factor 21 | Involved in suppressing the growth of lung cancer cells. |
| TS | Thymidylate synthase | Recent findings suggest that TS might be a biomarker for NSCLC treated with pemetrexed. |
| FGFR1 | Fibroblast Growth Factor Receptor, that mediates cell survival and proliferation. | Seen in ~7% of all non-small cell lung cancer adenocarcinoma patients. Gene amplification of FGFR1 has been detected in 13- 25% of squamous tumors. For patients with squamous cell carcinomas, FGFR1 amplification is associated with smoking and with worse overall survival. Ask your doctor about the LungMAP trial. |
| KRAS | One of RAS family of oncogenes, stands for Kirsten Rat Sarcoma gene, works with downstream effector genes to control cell proliferation and apoptosis | Activating KRAS mutations are observed in approximately 20 to 25 percent of lung adenocarcinomas in the United States and are generally associated with a history of smoking. Ask your doctor about clinical trials focusing on downstream effector inhibition, such as mTOR, MEK etc. |
| RET Fusions | RET protooncogene encodes Rearranged during transfection (RET) transmembrane receptor tyrosine kinase. | RET gene fusions occur in approximately 1- 2% of NSCLCs, typically in patients who are younger than age 60 years, former light smokers or never-smokers, with early lymph node metastasis and tumors that are poorly differentiated. |
| DDR2 | Discoidin Domain Receptor 2 | The DDR2 gene encodes a cell surface receptor tyrosine kinase that is mutated to an active form in about 4 percent of squamous cell carcinomas of the lung. Dasatinib might be a treatment option. Ask your doctor about clinical trials. |

Molecular testing will help your oncologist determine if the lung tumor is one of the four well-known genetic alterations that have an approved targeted drug (*EGFR*, *EGFR T790M*, *ROS1*, or *ALK*). If the testing is negative on all four genes, your oncologist may be able to enroll you in a clinical trial for another targeted therapy or may elect to treat you with other more traditional therapies. Much research is being done on other genetic mutations that may be treatable someday.

The use of Next Generation Sequencing (NGS) also called Comprehensive Genomic Profiling (CGP) is a deep dive look into the molecular makeup of your cancer regardless of cancer type and may help your doctor determine which clinical trial might be best for you. For more information on NGS, please visit Foundation Medicine, www.foundationmedicine.com. By the time you are reading this guidebook, researchers may have identified additional mutations. Please contact ALCF for more information or an updated list of molecular mutations.

*This Foundation is tenacious, innovative, collaborative and determined that lung cancer patients will no longer be left behind.*

*—Jaimi Julian Thompson*

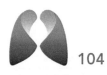

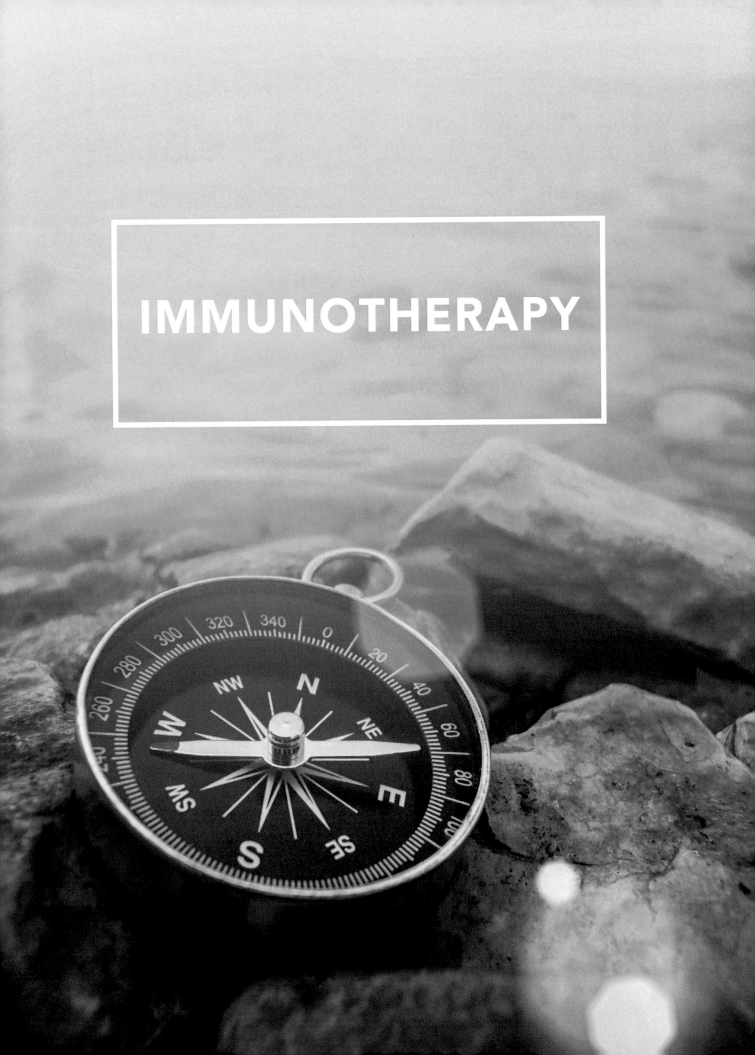

# IMMUNOTHERAPY

# IMMUNOTHERAPY FOR THE TREATMENT OF LUNG CANCER

## What is the immune system and how does it work?

- The immune system is a collection of unique cells and substances they produce, that act as the body's defense mechanism against infections and anything 'foreign.'

- Immune cells travel through the body and keep track of all cells and substances normally found in the body. These cells are trained to recognize pathogens like bacteria, viruses, etc. and abnormal cells in the body as 'foreign' and eliminate them.

- This process of recognition and elimination is based on the presence of molecules (such as proteins) on the surface of all cells that the immune cells use to distinguish between 'self' and foreign.

## What is Cancer Immunotherapy?

- Immunotherapy is a treatment modality that employs several different tricks to stimulate the patient's own immune system to fight their cancer.

- Cancer cells have devised unique ways to evade surveillance and elimination by the immune system by cloaking themselves to appear as normal cells.

- Immunotherapy aims to either *specifically* un-'cloak' these cancer cells and expose them to the immune system, OR, train the immune system to fight harder and smarter in a general, non-specific fashion.

- Immunotherapy holds great potential for treating cancer, as no other therapy can compare with the elaborate network of cellular interactions and pathways employed by the human body to rid itself of foreign entities.

**Immunotherapy has several advantages over chemotherapy and targeted therapy:**

Traditionally, lung cancer has not been considered an immune-responsive cancer given the very limited benefit seen with earlier immunotherapeutic agents such as bacille Calmette-Guerin vaccination, interleukin (IL)-2, interferons etc. However, recent data coming in on early phase clinical trials of various new immunotherapies for lung cancer show immense promise in terms of *response rates* and *survival advantages* that outweigh anything else currently available, typically adding months, if not years to life expectancy for lung cancer patients. However, these therapies are relatively new, still in the *experimental* stage (not FDA-approved) and there are several characteristics about patient selection for therapy, patient response, therapy resistance that we currently do not understand.

With that being said, immunotherapy has several advantages over chemotherapy and targeted therapy:

- Immunotherapy has demonstrated *a low toxicity profile* relative to chemotherapy and targeted therapy.
- Because the biological system is *sensitive* to even very minor alterations, the immune system can detect relatively low numbers of cancer cells and mount a response to eliminate them.
- The immune system has a strong *'memory,'* in that it remembers the foreign cells it was exposed to and each time it encounters those cells again, it gets activated and works to eliminate them. This immune memory bestows *longer lasting tumor control,* as against chemotherapy and targeted therapy that need to be constantly replenished in the body. Since immune responses

stimulated by immunotherapy, once generated, are always remembered by the body and activated each time cancer recurs, this therapeutic modality produces *durable, sustained tumor response.*

## What are the various types of immunotherapy effective for lung cancer?

There are currently three types of immunotherapies that are being evaluated to treat cancer, listed below.

1. Immune modulators such as Immune Checkpoint Inhibitors
2. Cancer Vaccines
3. Adoptive T cell Transfer

Three drugs belonging to the first category of Immune Checkpoint Inhibitors are now FDA-approved for use by patients with advanced, metastatic non-small cell lung cancer patients. These drugs are Nivolumab (Opdivo, manufactured by Bristol Myers Squibb), Pembrolizumab (Keytruda, manufactured by Merck) and Atezolizumab (Tecentriq, manufactured by Genentech).

## What are Immune Checkpoint Inhibitors?

- The main role of the immune system is to keep track of what is 'self' and, identify and eliminate anything that is 'foreign.'
- In order to prevent the immune system from attacking its own normal 'self' cells, the body has evolved several checks and balances that keep the immune system under control.
- These checks and balances are like the brakes in a car that prevent the car from going into overdrive, and are designed to prevent or abort actions that could be self-destructive.

- A breach in these systems results in the immune system recognizing normal cells as 'non-self' and eliminating them, resulting in auto-immune diseases like lupus and arthritis.
- Cancer cells have evolved ways and means to overtake these normal checkpoints, locally block the immune response in the vicinity of the tumor, and effectively escape detection and elimination by the immune system.
- Two immune checkpoints that have been targeted recently to lift the brakes from the immune system so that it goes full force to attack cancer cells are CTLA4 and PD-1/PDL1.
- Checkpoint inhibitors basically undo the local blockade of the immune response evoked by cancer cells and allow the immune system to resume normal function and attack the tumor.

## How do PD-1/PDL1 checkpoint inhibitors work?

- PD-1 stands for Programmed Death receptor-1.
- It is a protein expressed on the surface of immune cells, specifically T cells, a kind of white blood cells that fight infection and other foreign bodies.
- PD-1 interacts with a protein on the surface of normal cells of the body, PDL1 (Programmed Death Ligand 1).
- This PD1-PDL1 interaction is an immune checkpoint, i.e. a signal to the immune system to not mount an attack on the body's own cells.
- Cancer cells usurp this mechanism and express PDL1 on their surface to fool the immune system into believing that they are normal cells.
- Therefore, blocking the PD-1/ PDL1 interaction is the target for anti-cancer immunotherapy, as PD-1 or PDL1 inhibitors allow the immune system to then recognize the cancer cells as foreign and eliminate them.
- It is encouraging that lung cancer cells express PDL1 on their surface and are therefore amenable to PD-1 and PDL1 blockade.

- PD-1/ PDL1 *checkpoint inhibitors* are molecules that bind to either PD-1 (expressed on immune cells) or PDL1 (expressed on cancer cells) and block the surface of these proteins, preventing them from interacting with each other.

- The tolerability of these immune checkpoint inhibitors has been generally good, with few dose-limiting toxicities reported. The most common irAEs or immune related Adverse Events reported are: dermatologic (rash, pruritus, and vitiligo), gastrointestinal (diarrhea and colitis), endocrine (hypothyroidism and hyperthyroidism), and hepatic (hepatitis and increased liver function enzymes) events, as well as pneumonitis, uveitis, infusion-related events, and fatigue.

- A phase I trial designed to test the safety and clinical activity of an antibody that blocks PD-L1 found that around 25% of patients with non-small-cell lung cancer (NSCLC) responded to the drug. The results of this ongoing study reported at the 2014 American Society of Clinical Oncology (ASCO) meeting showed that this response rate is better than the 3% rate generally seen in patients who are receiving their third course of chemotherapy after earlier treatments have failed.

- **PD-1 vs. PDL1:** Although the response rates are similar for the inhibitors that bind to PD-1 on immune cells and those that block PD-L1 on tumor cells, early data suggest that there may be a slight safety advantage in targeting PD-L1. A phase I trial of a PD-1 inhibitor reported a 3% incidence of drug-related pneumonitis (inflammation of the lung tissue) but this side effect has so far been less severe or absent with the PD-L1 inhibitors.

- **Effects in smokers vs. non-smokers:** Early results suggest that both kinds of inhibitors-anti-PD1 and anti-PDL1- seem to benefit smokers more than non-smokers. Results of a phase I trial of a PD-L1 inhibitor presented at the 2013 European Cancer Congress indicated that 26% of smokers responded to the drug, but only 10% of never-smokers responded. Researchers speculate that this is probably due to the greater number of mutations present in smokers' tumors, an abundance that would probably present the newly awakened immune response with a far greater array of tumor antigens to respond to, and mount a response against.

## Which immunotherapeutic drugs are currently approved for the treatment of lung cancer?

Currently, three immunotherapy drugs are FDA-approved for the treatment of patients with advanced, metastatic non-small cell lung cancer, whose disease has progressed during or after platinum-based chemotherapy, or in some cases, targeted therapy.

Two of these drugs are anti-PD1 inhibitors- Nivolumab (Opdivo, manufactured by Bristol Myers Squibb) and Pembrolizumab (Keytruda, manufactured by Merck), and third drug is an anti-PDL1 inhibitor- Atezolizumab (Tecentriq, manufactured by Genentech). These immunotherapeutic drugs are proteins called monoclonal antibodies that bind specifically to either PD-1 (Nivolumab and Pembrolizumab) or PDL1 (Atezolizumab) and take the brakes off the immune system, so that it can mount a powerful and sustained response against a patients' tumors.

## What are the differences in the use of the three Immunotherapy drugs for Lung Cancer?

One differentiating factor between these three approved immunotherapy drugs (for non-small cell lung cancer patients that progress on first line therapies) is the need for

PDL1 companion diagnostic testing, i.e. testing for the presence of the protein PDL1 on patients' tumors. Treatment by Nivolumab or atezolizumab does not require PDL1 testing, while treatment by Pembrolizumab does.

Pembrolizumab use requires initial testing for the presence of the protein PDL1 on a patient's tumors, by an FDA-approved companion diagnostic test- the immunohistochemistry (IHC) test called the PDL1 IHC 22C3 pharmDx test. This is the first companion diagnostic test that has been approved to check for the expression/ presence of the PDL1 protein in NSCLC tumors. This is an important advance, because the use of the companion diagnostic test will potentially help to identify NSCLC patients most likely to respond to this therapy and benefit from it. This companion diagnostic test is made commercially available to laboratories in the U.S. through Dako North America Inc., and testing using the assay is available at U.S. reference laboratories including Laboratory Corporation of America® Holdings (LabCorp®), Quest Diagnostics, and GE Healthcare Clarient Diagnostic Services.

Another difference between the use of Nivolumab, Pembrolizumab and Atezolizumab is the schedules of administration and dosing of the drugs. Pembrolizumab has been approved for administration every 3 weeks at 2mg/kg intravenously over 30 minutes, while Nivolumab has been approved for use every 2 weeks at 3 mg/kg intravenously, over 60 minutes. The most recently approved drug, Atezolizumab, has been approved for use every 3 weeks at 1200 mg as an intravenous infusion over 60 minutes.

The third difference, as mentioned earlier, is that Nivolumab and Pembrolizumab are anti-PD1 medicines, while Atezolizumab is an anti-PDL1 medicine. It is not clear if one drug is better than the other, and the decision to go on any one of these should be made in consultation with your physician.

## What are the side effects of treatment with Immunotherapeutic drugs?

Most common side effects observed in the clinical trials that evaluated these three immunotherapeutic agents for lung cancer patients were fatigue, decreased appetite, dyspnea, and cough. However, it is important to note that immunotherapeutic agents may be associated with immune-mediated side effects in the lungs, colon and hormone-producing glands. Immune-mediated adverse reactions observed with these drugs in clinical trials have included pneumonitis, colitis, hepatitis, hypophysitis, hyperthyroidism, hypothyroidism, type 1 diabetes mellitus, and nephritis. Based on the severity of the adverse reaction, these immunotherapeutic drugs should either be withheld or discontinued and corticosteroids should be administered.

## How can I access an immunotherapy drug for my lung cancer?

The manufacturers of all three immunotherapeutic drugs currently approved for lung cancer have financial assistance programs to ensure patients have access to these promising medicines.

Merck has programs that ensure patients who are prescribed Pembrolizumab have access to the therapy. The Merck Access Program provides reimbursement support for eligible patients receiving Pembrolizumab, including help with out-of-pocket costs and co-pay assistance. Merck also offers financial assistance for eligible patients who are uninsured through their patient assistance program. More information is available by calling 1-855-257-3932 or visiting www.merckaccessprogram-keytruda.com.

Nivolumab is marketed by Bristol Myers Squibb (BMS). BMS Access Support®, the Bristol-Myers Squibb Reimbursement Services program, is designed to support access to BMS medicines and expedite time to therapy through reimbursement support as well as assistance for patient out-of-pocket costs. More information about our reimbursement support services can be obtained by calling 1-800-861-0048 or by visiting www.bmsaccesssupport.com.

Atezolizumab is manufactured by Genentech. Access Solutions is part of Genentech's commitment to helping people access the Genentech medicines they are prescribed, regardless of their ability to pay. The team of in-house specialists at Access Solutions is dedicated to helping people navigate the access and reimbursement process, and to providing assistance to eligible patients in the United States who are uninsured or cannot afford the out-of-pocket costs for their medicine. To date, the team has helped more than 1.4 million patients access the medicines they need. Please contact **Access Solutions (866) 4ACCESS/(866) 422-2377** or visit http://www.Genentech-Access.com for more information.

## What is CTLA 4?

- CTLA4 stands for Cytotoxic T Lymphocyte Antigen 4.
- It is expressed on immune cells, such as the T cells, and plays a major role in activating immune response.
- **Ipilimumab (Yervoy®)** is the first checkpoint inhibitor that was approved by the FDA for the treatment of metastatic melanoma. It is currently being evaluated to treat other solid tumors like lung and renal cancer.
- Ipilimumab is a monoclonal antibody which targets the CTLA-4 checkpoint on activated immune cells, and has been approved for use in other cancers such as melanoma.

- Ipilimumab is currently in clinical trials for the treatment of lung cancer patients. Contact your physician or the Addario Lung Cancer Foundation to learn more about these clinical trials, and how you can participate.

- **Tremelimumab,** another antibody targeting the CTLA-4 molecule, is being tested in a phase II clinical trial for patients with mesothelioma and lung cancer.

## What is Combination Therapy?

- Combination therapy is combining one or more different therapeutics for increased efficacy and tumor shrinkage, such that the effects of the combination are greater than the effects produced by sum of the parts.

- Combining two different therapeutics may be sequential (one after the other) or concurrent (both therapies administered together).

- Studies are underway to understand if and how immunotherapy may be combined with chemotherapy and/or radiotherapy. These studies are based on the hypotheses that the antigens released from dying cancer cells upon effective chemotherapy, may serve to stimulate the immune system, mount a tumor-specific immune response, and thereby enhance the efficacy of the immunotherapeutic.

- A combination of the immune checkpoint inhibitor Ipilimumab with chemotherapy has shown encouraging results in both small cell and non-small cell lung cancer.

## Combination immune checkpoint approaches

- Studies are also underway to evaluate dual checkpoint blockade to increase the proportion and durability of tumor responses.

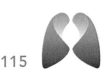

- Early evidence suggests that combination strategies that involve immune checkpoint blockade may have additive effects in the clinic.

- In patients with advanced melanoma, combination therapy with nivolumab and Ipilimumab showed preliminary activity much greater than that seen in previous experience with either agent alone: 40% of patients on a concurrent regimen had an objective response, and 65% had evidence of clinical activity.

- Ongoing trials in lung cancer exploring combinatorial checkpoint blockade will provide further insight into the use of these new therapies for lung cancer patients.

- New data from immunotherapy studies points to the fact that combining immune checkpoint inhibitors holds the potential to improve therapeutic efficacy.

## What are cancer vaccines?

- A vaccine is typically a biological agent used to stimulate and train the immune system to recognize this agent as 'foreign', mount a response to eliminate it from the body, and create 'memory' such that if the agent is encountered again, the body readily clears it from the system.

- Vaccines may be either *prophylatic* (they prevent future infection by the agent) or *therapeutic* (they treat current infections).

- Cancer vaccines are therapeutic. These vaccines use proteins expressed on the surface of cancer cells to train the immune system to recognize tumors and destroy them.

- So far, there is only one FDA-approved vaccine for cancer: Provenge approved for the treatment of advanced prostate cancer in April 2010.

- There is excitement around the use of cancer vaccines for lung cancer as lung tumors over-express specific proteins such as MAGE-3 (overexpressed in 42% of all lung cancers, 35% early stage and 55% late stage NSCLCs), NY-ESO-1 (overexpressed in 30% of all lung cancers), p53 (overexpressed in 50% of lung cancers), survivin, MUC-1, etc., which can serve as agents to train the immune system to recognize these proteins on cancer cells and specifically kill those cells.

## What is Adoptive T Cell Transfer?

- The third major type of immunotherapy currently being evaluated for lung cancer is adoptive T Cell transfer which is a process that involves 1) removing a patient's immune cells, specifically the T cells from their body, 2) treating these cells with various chemicals and other biological factors in a lab dish such that they recognize antigens on tumors and mount a strong immune response, and 3) re-inject these activated immune cells back into the patient's body.

## Patient response to cancer immunotherapy

- One of the challenges of immunotherapy for lung cancer is the variability in patient response: while some patients see very durable and lasting responses, others only get a partial response to the therapy and progress, while others see no response at all.
- Studies are underway to understand the underlying reasons for these differences in response to immunotherapy in lung cancer patients. These studies will hopefully uncover biomarkers of response to these therapies that can be used to better select patients who are most

likely to respond, while sparing toxicity and side effects in those unlikely to respond, thereby allow tailoring therapy to patients based on the specifics of their cancer.

• Since immunotherapies are designed to stimulate the immune system, these agents are not suited for patients that have a history of autoimmune disorders or previous immunosuppressive therapy.

## The Future Holds Promise

Immunotherapy holds promise to be a critical component in the care of lung cancer patients across the spectrum, all the way from neoadjuvant, adjuvant, and maintenance therapy. Its ability to unlock the patient's own immune system and stimulate it to eradicate cancer has immense potential that is only now beginning to be understood. With that being said, there are still several mechanistic and clinical unknowns that are currently being evaluated to fully utilize these therapies in a way that's best suited for lung cancer patients.

## Ongoing studies are currently evaluating:

• The use of immunotherapies earlier in the treatment journey. The three immunotherapeutic drugs currently approved for lung cancer patients have been approved for use in the second line setting, i.e. for patients that have received either chemotherapy or targeted therapies, and have progressed during or on these treatments. Current clinical trials underway are evaluating the use of immunotherapeutic agents for treating newly diagnosed lung cancer patients, upfront, in the front-line setting. Early data from these clinical trials show that Pembrolizumab has promising activity in newly diagnosed lung cancer patients whose tumors express PDL1 (greater than 50%). These early data show that monotherapy with anti-PD1 checkpoint inhibitors in the front line setting might be best served in patients that are PDL1-positive.

- Also under current evaluation are combinations of immunotherapeutic agents with other kinds of therapies, such as chemotherapy, radiation therapy and targeted therapies. These combinations are currently in clinical trials. Contact the Bonnie J. Addario Lung Cancer Foundation at portal@lungcancerfoundation.org to find out how you can participate in these trials, and access these treatments.

1. Immunotherapy + Chemotherapy: The rationale for the combinations is clear. Chemotherapy will kill cancer cells, causing the release of cancer antigens or proteins inside the cancer cell, which get exposed to the immune system. With the immunotherapy drugs, the immune system is now primed to mount a response to these antigens for a meaningful and deeper response. Early data from the combination of Pembrolizumab with chemotherapy in newly diagnosed, previously never treated patients show that this combination is effective even in patients whose tumors do not express high levels of PDL1.

2. Immunotherapy + Immunotherapy: Combinations of two different immunotherapeutic agents are being evaluated for lung cancer patients, such as combination of anti-PD1 Nivolumab and anti-CTLA4 Ipilimumab. This combination has been approved for the treatment of melanoma patients and is showing promise for lung cancer patients. A word of caution on the use of combinations of immunotherapies is the potential increase in side effects of the two immunotherapeutic agents.

3. Immunotherapy + Radiation Therapy: For several years we have known about an interesting phenomenon with RT called the abscopal effect

(ab-scopus, away from target) where we see tumor regression in lesions distant from the targeted site. Now RT also release antigens from dying cancer cells that can prime the immune system to mount an attack. Combining RT with immunotherapy therefore holds potential, as release of antigens combined with a primed immune system that has its 'brakes' removed will form the perfect storm to completely wipe out the tumor. This hypothesis is currently being tested in several clinical trials for lung cancer patients.

4.     Immunotherapy + Targeted Therapy: These combinations are one of the ways in which we can convert 'cold' tumors that do not respond to immunotherapies (because these tumors do not have enough immune cells in the tumor microenvironment, also called 'immune deserts') to 'hot' tumors. There is emerging data to support that some targeted therapies can increase the influx of immune cells (T cells) into the tumor microenvironment, and combining these with the immunotherapeutic agent makes sure that these cells mount an attack against the tumor.

- The most appropriate dose and duration of immunotherapy.

- Where immunotherapies stand in the lung cancer treatment continuum, what the optimal timing is for their administration, depending on tumor load and the stage of the disease. Can we re-administer immunotherapeutic agents after responders progress? If we do re-administer, should it be just with a single agent or a combination? What is the optimal duration?

- The variations in patient response to immunotherapy (why some patients respond while others do not, why do some patients have durable responses that last while others relapse quickly), such that these therapeutics can be tailored to patients based on the underlying specifics of their disease.

- Specific biomarkers for patient selection and disease response.

- Mechanisms of immune resistance and post-immunotherapy relapse strategies employed by the cancer.

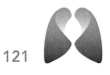

*Why do we support the Addario Lung Cancer Foundation? Because they are compassionate, cost-effective and patient focused. There is not enough research, but this awesome and poignant video is worth watching about a group of Lung Cancer patients who self-organized and got the Addario Lung Cancer Foundation to do a rare cancer study of their specific (ROS1) mutation. It is just beautiful and represents hope.*

https://vimeopro.com/
lungcancerfoundation/gala/
video/191728298

—Ron Fong

# SMALL CELL LUNG CANCER TREATMENTS

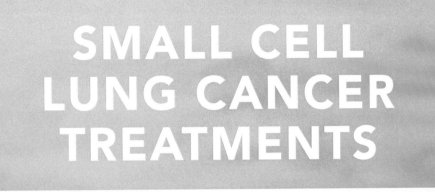

*Educated and empowered
patients do much better.*

*—Bonnie J. Addario, survivor*

# SMALL CELL
# LUNG CANCER – TREATMENTS

## Overview

Small cell lung cancer (SCLC) is the other type of lung cancer. Although it is less common than non-small cell lung cancer (NSCLC), SCLC grows and spreads through the body early in the disease – sometimes before any symptoms are noticed. Of all lung cancers, only about 10 to 15% are SCLC and almost all of these cases are found in people who currently smoke or have smoked cigarettes.[2] Because of the connection with cigarette smoking, SCLC is a little more common in men than in women. In addition, SCLC is usually described as *limited* or *extensive.*

SCLC is called "limited stage" when the total area involved by the disease can be targeted with one radiation field. This means that small cell lung cancer can still be limited stage if it moves to lymph nodes in the middle of the chest known as the mediastinum. Most importantly, having limited stage disease means you can be treated with curative intent. "Extensive stage" SCLC is cancer that has spread outside of one radiation field and usually means the disease cannot be cured, only controlled for a period of time.

SCLC typically starts in the bronchi (large breathing tubes) located behind the breastbone in the middle of the chest. True to the name, the cells in SCLC are smaller than the cells in NSCLC; however, because these cells grow very quickly, the tumors they create can be larger than NSCLC tumors. This type of lung cancer also tends to metastasize rapidly, or spread to other areas of the body, such as the brain, liver, or bones faster than NSCLC in most cases.

125

## How is SCLC treated?

Chemotherapy is the main treatment for small cell lung cancers. Since SCLC may spread before you notice any symptoms, removing the lung tumor by surgery rarely cures the cancer. Even when surgery is used to treat SCLC, it is never the only treatment you will receive. Laser treatments and experimental treatments available in a clinical trial may also be used to treat SCLC.

### Surgery

Surgery is rarely used to treat SCLC and if it is, it is rarely the <u>only</u> treatment since the cancer has typically spread before it is diagnosed. Your thoracic surgeon may also use one of the surgical techniques, previously described, to obtain tissue to determine the type of cancer and how far it has spread.

### Chemotherapy

Since SCLC tends to travel outside of the lung, chemotherapy treatments are designed to kill cancer cells that have metastasized into other areas of the body. Taken by mouth or injected into a vein, there are many different types of chemotherapy that your oncologist may prescribe for you. Most often, a platinum-based drug such as cisplatin or carboplatin is coupled with etoposide, which has been found to be most effective treatment for limited or extensive stage small cell lung cancer.

Additional chemotherapy drugs that have been approved for treatment of small cell lung cancer are included in the following table:

| Approved for | Generic Name | Brand Name(s) |
|---|---|---|
| Both NSCLC & SCLC | Carboplatin | Paraplat, Paraplatin® |
| Both NSCLC & SCLC | Cisplatin | Platinol®, Platinol A-Q |
| Both NSCLC & SCLC | Docetaxel | Taxotere® |
| Both NSCLC & SCLC | Etoposide | Toposar®, VePesid® |
| SCLC | Etoposide Phosphate | Etopophos® |
| Both NSCLC & SCLC | Gemcitabine Hydrochloride | Gemzar® |
| Both NSCLC & SCLC | Ifosfamide | Ifex® |
| SCLC | Methotrexate | Abitrexate, Folex®, Folex PFS, Methotrexate LPF, Mexate®, Mexate A-Q |
| Both NSCLC & SCLC | Paclitaxel | Taxol® |
| Both NSCLC & SCLC | Topotecan Hydrochloride | Hycamtin® |
| Both NSCLC & SCLC | Vinblastine | Velban™ |

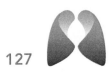

## Radiation Therapy

For SCLC, your oncologist may prescribe radiation treatments. Treatment with radiation may also help to relieve symptoms such as breathing problems. Your team may use many different types of radiation therapies to treat your SCLC. Radiation treatments are usually used in a treatment plan with chemotherapy.

> Monthly infusions of zoledronic acid (Zometa®) or subcutaneous injections of denosumab (Xgeva®) are used in patients with bone metastases to prevent new bone lesions from forming and to help heal existing bone lesions.

## Treatment for limited SCLC

If you are diagnosed with limited SCLC, the first option might be surgery if the tumor is small. However, it is more likely that you will be started on a combination of chemotherapy and radiation therapy.

About 50% of people with SCLC will develop metastases to the brain during their cancer journey.[19] Your oncologist may also prescribe *prophylactic cranial irradiation* (PCI) to prevent spread of the cancer to your brain. PCI is a kind of radiation treatment that may be used to kill cancer cells in the brain that may not be visible on x-rays or scans.

## Treatment for extensive SCLC

If you are diagnosed with extensive SCLC, chemotherapy will usually be the first-line of treatment prescribed by your oncologist. If the tumor shrinks, your doctor will usually prescribe prophylactic cranial irradiation (PCI) treatments

> Talk to your oncologist about the possibility of participating in a clinical trial.

to prevent metastasis to the brain. PCI is a kind of radiation treatment that may be used to kill cancer cells in the brain that may not be visible on x-rays or scans. Your oncologist may recommend a clinical trial as a course of treatment. Clinical trials are studies that have shown enough promise that they are now being done on humans. See the Clinical Trials chapter for more information on how to find clinical trials in your area.

### Treatment for recurrent SCLC

Even with aggressive treatment, small cell lung cancer may come back or *recur*. It is a type of cancer that responds extremely well to radiation and chemotherapy in most cases. The problem is that the responses generally do not last very long and are not "durable."

When the diagnosis of SCLC is made, you should discuss with your healthcare team the treatment plan you prefer such as chemotherapy and/or radiation. The plan may include treatment of the disease or symptom management (see the Transitional Care Planning section in the Living with Lung Cancer chapter for further discussion of treatment plans).

*We're very fortunate to
have the Foundation and it's been
our saving grace. It really has been.
It is giving us hope and they
keep us going every day for
our mom.*

*—Yvette, caregiver*

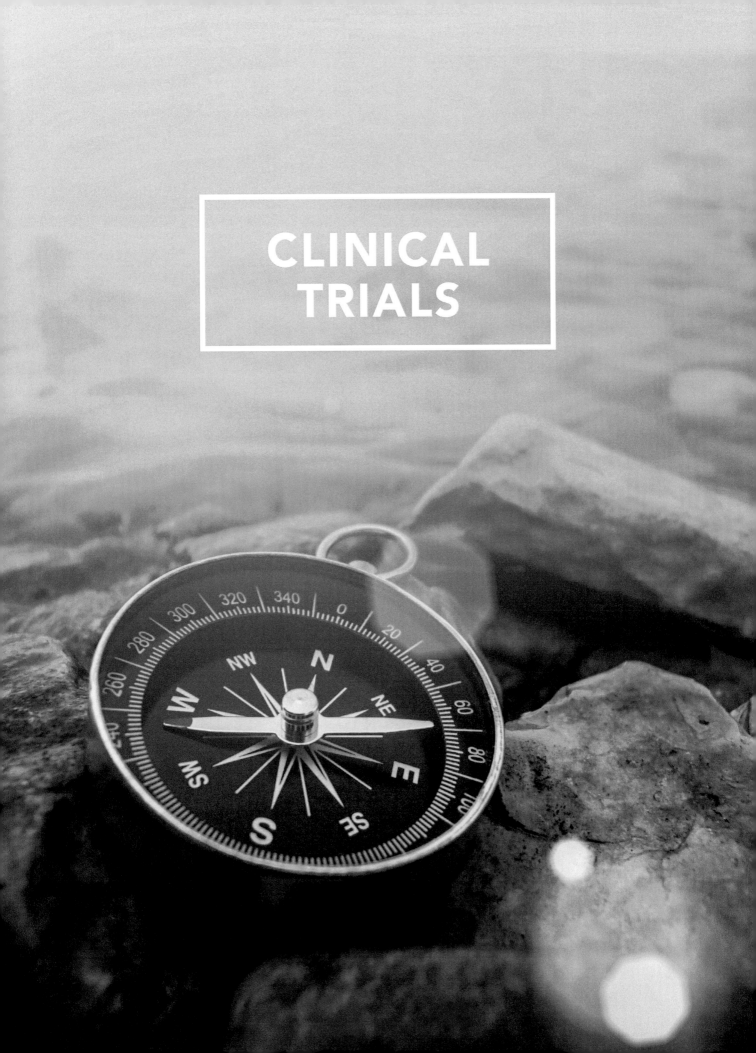

# CLINICAL
# TRIALS

*I really appreciate the Foundation, all the work they've done and the guidance they've given me.*

*—Robert, survivor*

# CLINICAL TRIALS

## What are Clinical Trials?

"A clinical trial provides the means by which your doctors can evaluate an important scientific question relating to your cancer. In most cases, the question of interest is whether a new drug or novel treatment approach is better than an existing treatment or at least worthy of further evaluation." Paul Hesketh, MD, Lahey Clinical Medical Center. A clinical trial is a research study that has progressed from a scientific question through laboratory testing and is now ready for human volunteers. Clinical trials are critical to the development of new lung cancer treatments, ways to ease the symptoms of lung cancer treatments, and collect tumor or blood samples for research. These new treatments may include drugs, surgical procedures, and new ways to manage side effects. The clinical trials process is overseen by the Food and Drug Administration (FDA), a local institutional review board (also known as an ethics committee), and a physician specifically trained to manage clinical trials.

A clinical trial may be referred to as a "research study," "study," or "trial." The team

Questions to ask your oncologist and healthcare team about the clinical trial you are considering:

- What do you hope to learn from this clinical trial?
- Has the experimental treatment/procedure been studied before?
- What phase is this clinical trial?
- Who will be in charge of my care during the trial?
- Will my care change based upon my response to the treatment during the trial?
- What are the risks and benefits?
- How long will the trial last?
- Who pays for the trial?
- Will my insurance cover the treatment?
- Will I be paid?
- Can I be forced or asked to leave the trial?
- Can I learn the results of the trial?

that manages the clinical trial is often referred to as the "clinical trials team," "research staff," or "study staff." Do not let the names confuse you as they all mean the same thing.

## What types of clinical trials might be available?

There are several types of clinical trials for which you might be eligible. Your eligibility for any trial will be based on very specific requirements, so it is important you discuss these requirements with your oncologist and the study staff. Clinical trials may be classified as:

- Prevention trials – Prevention trials explore factors that may increase or decrease your risk of developing lung cancer.
- Screening trials – Screening trials develop new and better ways to detect cancer.
- Diagnostic trials – Diagnostic trials develop better tests or procedures for diagnosing cancer.
- Treatment trials – When most people think of clinical trials, treatment trials are the ones that most often come to mind. Treatment trials evaluate specific medications, radiation treatments, and new surgical techniques to treat cancer.
- Supportive care trials – Supportive care trials, or quality-of-life trials, evaluate medications, radiation treatments, and new surgical techniques to decrease symptoms of cancer or the side effects of cancer treatments.

## What are Clinical Trial phases?

In order for a new drug to be approved by the Food and Drug Administration (FDA) for use in humans, the drug must pass through a rigorous testing process. This testing process is called a clinical trial and is composed of four different phases usually referred to as phases I through IV.

Phase I trials are the first level in which the researchers evaluate safety, determine safe amount of drug and identify side effects that might occur with the treatment. Before this phase, the treatment has already been researched at length in the lab and on animals and the drug has been determined to be ready for use in humans. The research team will adjust the amount of the treatment you receive at different intervals in the trial while monitoring the treatment's side effects. Typically, there may be only 20 to 80 people selected to participate in a phase I clinical trial.

Phase II trials begin after a treatment has been found to be safe in phase I trials. During phase II, the research team will use a specific treatment, or combination of treatments, to determine the effectiveness for a specific type of cancer. A phase II clinical trial may include 100 to 300 people.

Phase III trials will be done when a treatment is found to be effective in phase II trials. During this phase, the treatment will be tested on a large number of patients comparing standard treatments (treatment you receive outside of the clinical trial) with the new treatment. If you participate in a phase III clinical trial, you may be randomly assigned to a control or test group. If you are assigned to the control group, you will receive the standard treatment for your specific type and stage of lung cancer. If you are assigned to the test group, you will receive the new treatment. Results from the two groups will be closely monitored by the research team to determine which treatment is most effective and the side effects of the treatment. Phase III trials include up to 3,000 patients.

Phase IV trials begin after the treatment has been approved by the FDA. In phase IV clinical trials, the treatment will be given to a much larger group of patients. In this phase, additional information will be gathered about effectiveness, side effects that might not have been previously identified, and safety issues that can only be identified in a larger group of participants.

## How can I learn about the purpose, risk and benefits of a clinical trial?

Informed consent is the process of learning the facts about the clinical trial before deciding whether you want to participate. To help you decide whether to participate, the doctors and nurses involved in the trial, called the study staff, will explain the details of the trial. The study staff will provide you with an informed consent document that includes details about the trial: its purpose, length of time the clinical trial will be open, any required procedures, and the key contacts. The study staff will outline all of the potential risks and benefits in the informed consent document. After understanding all of the information, you will decide whether to sign the document. Informed consent is not a contract, and you will be able to withdraw from the trial at any time. The study staff should provide updated information to you throughout the trial.

> "When I speak to patients about clinical trials, I always review the clinical benefits of participating in the trial. But I also say, the potential advantages of participating in a clinical trial include: 1) gaining access to a new treatment approach not otherwise available; 2) providing your doctors greater insights into your cancer; 3) helping to generate knowledge that may help future cancer patients. Ask your doctor if a clinical trial is available to you."
> – Paul Hesketh, MD, Lahey Clinic Medical Center

## What are the potential benefits of clinical trials?

Participating in a clinical trial may have several potential benefits for you. By participating in the trial, you will:

* Play an active role in determining the direction of your health care
* Have access to new treatments before they are widely available
* Receive expert medical care at leading health care facilities
* Help others by contributing to medical research

## What are the risks of clinical trials?

Before you agree to participate in a clinical trial, you should talk to your oncologist and the doctor in charge of the trial to make sure you understand the possible risks. You should understand that the treatment being used may not be better and side effects may be worse than the standard treatment. Because the treatment is new, your healthcare team may not know all of the side effects that you will experience. A clinical trial may require more time and attention from your healthcare team and from you than would a non-clinical trial treatment regimen. This extra time may include trips to the cancer center, more treatments, hospital stays and complex dosage requirements.

## When do I ask my healthcare team about participating in a clinical trial?

In a study done in 1999, the American Society of Clinical Oncologists found that only 3% of adults with cancer participate in clinical trials.[20] This low level of participation in clinical trials means that advances in cancer care do not happen as quickly as they might. Your participation in clinical trials can help to develop new cancer treatments f or all cancer patients.

Any time you are facing a treatment decision, you should ask about clinical trials that might be appropriate for you. Clinical trials are not just for advanced stage lung cancer – clinical trials are available for all stages of lung cancer. Ideally, your entire healthcare team will be available to talk to you about new treatments that may be available. For example, your oncologist, radiologist, and surgeon may each have access to information about different clinical trials. Once you know about clinical trials that might be appropriate, you should discuss the options with your entire team who can help you understand the benefits and risks based on your specific lung cancer and health status.

## Who takes care of me while I am in a clinical trial?

When you participate in a clinical trial, your healthcare needs and treatments will be managed by the clinical trial doctor (who may or may not be your oncologist) and the study staff (research nurse, research coordinator, laboratory personnel). This team will manage your care throughout your participation in the clinical trial.

The clinical trial and study staff is overseen by the Institutional Review Board (IRB) at the hospital, research facility, or cancer center. The role of the IRB is to make sure the trial is safe and is being managed properly. Typically, you will find that you will receive a very high quality of care while participating in a clinical trial because the study staff will closely monitor your condition while you participate in the trial.

## How long does a clinical trial last?

The length of clinical trials will vary based upon the research being studied. Some trials such as a tissue or blood collection trial may only involve a single visit. Other trials may last several years such as might occur in the case of a treatment trial. The informed consent form will detail the length of the clinical trial and should include how often you will be required to go to doctor visits, treatments, and follow up procedures.

Participating in a clinical trial is a commitment on your part. That said, you have the right to stop participating in a clinical trial at any time. Your clinical trial doctor may end your participation as well if the treatment is found to be unsafe, ineffective, if the clinical trial closes (research is complete) or for any other reason they deem appropriate. Be sure to understand your responsibilities in the clinical trial before you agree to participate.

## What does it cost to participate in a clinical trial?

Clinical trials are a critical part of cancer care. Most of the time, if you enroll in a clinical trial, the cost of tests, procedures, drugs, extra doctor visits, and any research related to the trial will be covered by the agency or company that sponsors the clinical trial. The sponsor may be a government agency, a college or university, a medical center, a non-profit organization, a drug company, or another private company.

Your health insurance plan may say that your participation in a clinical trial is "experimental" or "investigational." In this case, your insurance may not cover the costs of routine care including doctor visits, hospital stays, and tests or treatments that you would have normally received. Many states have laws in place regarding insurance coverage for clinical trials. Ask your study staff and your insurance company about the costs <u>before</u> you participate.

## How can I find clinical trials?

There are over 2,500 clinical trials in the US available to the lung cancer community at the time this guidebook was printed.[21] However, not all clinical trials will be available in your area. Clinical trials may be open at only one cancer center; others may be open in hundreds of cancer centers across the country. The number of participating centers depends on the disease being studied, the phase of the clinical trial, and the complexity of the clinical trial.

If you are interested in participating in a clinical trial, there are many sources of information. The two best sources of information are

• Your healthcare team (e.g. oncologist, radiologist, pulmonologist, etc.) – Ask your healthcare team if a clinical trial is appropriate for you at this time and what clinical trials are available at your center. If no trials are available at your center, ask your oncologist which investigation drugs or procedures might be right for you. With this information, you can search the government database for clinical trials in your area.

- U.S. National Institutes of Health (NIH) website of clinical trials located at http://ClinicalTrials.gov. There are many other internet sites with information on clinical trials, but these sites are generally built on information from the NIH website. This website lists both federally funded and privately supported clinical trials.

The NIH clinical trial list includes over 136,000 clinical trials available worldwide not just in the US. When you access the site, search for a clinical trial using the most specific information you have. For example, if your diagnosis is small cell lung cancer, search for "SCLC in the US." A list will open showing all of the studies that are in the database. In the listing, you will be able to tell the status of the clinical trial (Completed, Recruiting, Not yet Recruiting, Active, etc.). The list will include what conditions are being targeted in the trial and what treatments are actually being tested (drug, radiation therapy, etc.). Clicking on the name of the study will open a new window that shows extensive information about the specific study including how long the trial is expected to last, eligibility requirements, how outcomes will be measured and contacts for the trial. <u>If you find clinical trials that may be applicable to you, it is critical that you discuss them with your healthcare team.</u>[21]

> Searching for clinical trials may be very confusing since the resulting list may contain hundreds of possibilities. We are here to help—contact ALCF for assistance with identifying clinical trials in your area that may be of interest to you.

# WHO ARE CLINICAL TRIALS FOR: GUINEA PIGS, TEST PILOTS OR PRIZE POODLES?

BY D. ROSS CAMIDGE, MD, PhD

Director, Thoracic Oncology
Clinical and Clinical Research
Programs and Attending
Physician within the
Developmental Therapeutics
Program, University of Colorado
Cancer Center
Aurora, Colorado

# TABLE OF CONTENTS

## 1) Introduction:

While everyone with a diagnosis of cancer wants to get the best treatment, how does anyone know what the 'best' is?

A hundred years ago, when a salesman would stand on the back of a wagon and hold up a bottle of snake-oil, the 'best' medicine, at least at first, was often the one associated with the grandest sounding story of its discovery, or with the most impressive (paid) testimonials from those it had miraculously healed. Sadly, we still have snake-oil salesmen even in the twenty-first century. Although, these days they tend to operate from the Internet rather than the back of a wagon. Fortunately, we are not dependent on them as our sole source of information. Instead, over many years, a rigorous, evidence-based process for establishing and justifying the claims associated with any licensed medical product has evolved—a process involving the participation of patients in formalized clinical trials.

In this article I aim to explain why and how such clinical trials are performed in oncology. However, even if we recognize the value of objective data from clinical trials, this is, of course, not the same as automatically wanting to be a participant in the process yourself. Therefore, I also aim to give you some tips to help you and your family/friends decide on whether a particular trial is something that you, personally, should consider entering into at any stage of your cancer treatment journey.

## 2) Defining our cancer treatment terminology from the outset—stages of disease and lines of therapy:

Cancers come in all varieties, and in all shapes and sizes. Treatment for cancer ranges from surgery to radiotherapy to drug-based treatments—either on their own or as combinations of the different approaches. When a cancer has not spread very far around the body, perhaps only to the nearest set of lymph nodes that cover a given area of the body, or to no lymph nodes at all, it is usually referred to as an early stage cancer (this usually includes what is formally referred to as stage I or stage II cancer). If many different lymph nodes, or lymph nodes that are further away from the cancer, are involved, the cancer may be called locally advanced (this comprises most of what is called stage III disease). If the cancer has spread to other organs or structures in the body, such as the liver, bones or brain, then the cancer is considered even more advanced, and it is then usually called 'metastatic' or stage IV disease.

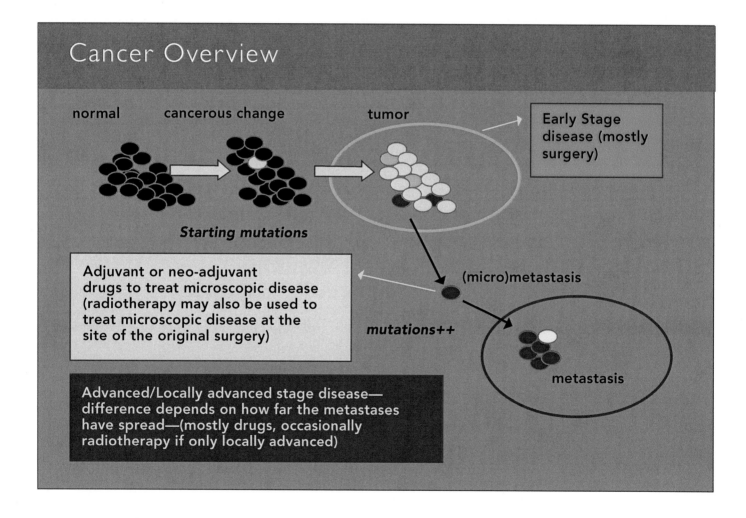

## 2a) Early Stage cancers:

In general, early stage cancers tend to be the most curable. The definitive treatment for these cancers is surgery, although high-dose radiotherapy, sometimes called radical radiotherapy, may be just as good in some situations. However, as most of us would rather have the cancer out of our bodies completely, radiotherapy, as an alternative to surgery for early stage disease, is usually reserved for those not fit enough for surgery or for those who don't wish surgery for other reasons. Chemotherapy, other drug-based treatments, radiotherapy or any combination of these is sometimes given before an operation. This is called 'neo-adjuvant' treatment and is usually to help shrink larger cancers down, either to make the operation easier and/or to increase the chances of getting rid of the cancer completely. Instead of, or in addition to, any neo-adjuvant treatment, **after** the operation a defined course of chemotherapy and sometimes radiotherapy (to the site of where the cancer once was) may also be given to reduce the chances of the cancer coming back. This is to treat microscopic disease that may be there, but that is too small to be detectable at the time. This is usually reserved for cancers with a higher risk of recurrence based on all of the available information after the cancer has been removed. This kind of 'insurance policy' approach, trying to maximize the chances of cure by giving extra therapies after an operation is called 'adjuvant' treatment.

## 2b) Locally advanced cancers:

While some locally advanced cancers may be removable by surgery, with or without the benefit of any associated neo-adjuvant and/or adjuvant treatments, other stage III cancers cannot be operated on. For example, in non-small cell lung cancer—one of the most common serious cancers—this is usually because the cancer has spread to involve lymph nodes on both sides of the middle of the chest, or to the lymph nodes

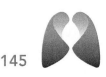

behind the collarbones. However, the exact location of the lymph nodes that distinguish between stage II (early stage disease) and stage III (locally advanced disease) will vary depending on the particular type of cancer and the part of the body affected. For cancers starting in the pelvis, like prostate or ovarian cancer, the lymph nodes that determine how far the cancer has spread will be very different from, for example, those relevant to a breast cancer that starts up in your chest wall.

Operations for locally advanced cancers have traditionally not been undertaken, although there are exceptions. This is because the risks of not removing all known deposits of the disease and of there being hidden metastatic disease in other parts of the body are considered to be very high for cancers that are locally advanced. Surgeons usually don't want to put patients through a large operation that will ultimately not cure them. Instead, a combination of high-dose radiotherapy to all known sites of disease, complemented by chemotherapy, is currently considered the standard of care for most inoperable stage III disease. The chemotherapy in this setting acts both to make the radiotherapy more effective and to treat any hidden microscopic disease in other parts of the body. Although some patients with stage III disease can be cured by this approach, the relapse rate is unfortunately still very high.

**2c) Advanced/metastatic cancers:**

In contrast to both early stage and locally advanced disease, advanced or metastatic disease is usually not treated with either surgery or high-dose radiotherapy, except under rare circumstances when there are very few sites involved (so-called 'oligometastatic disease'). Instead, when the disease is in multiple different places in the body, or in other areas difficult to localize precisely (for example, in fluid around the lungs), drugs, such as chemotherapy, that can circulate around many different places, are the mainstay of treatment. Treatment in this setting is not usually considered curative; instead it acts as a means to control the cancer. Control in this setting means several different things. For example, a slowing of the cancer's progress or a reduction in the amount of cancer in the body, for example shrinkage in the size of any masses seen on scans. Control may also mean an improvement in symptoms, if symptoms are present at the start of treatment. It may also mean a change in the natural history of the disease such that an individual with an incurable serious cancer lives longer. This sometimes can be very difficult to comprehend as a treatment goal. If you can't cure me —why even bother? Aren't you just dragging out the inevitable? There are two answers to these important questions. The first is purely pragmatic—if you have symptoms from the cancer and a treatment can improve these, or postpone their development, no matter how much time you have left it will be better quality time. However, there may be side effects associated with anti-cancer treatments and their severity and duration will always have to be weighed against the symptoms associated with the disease they are designed to treat. Pure symptomatic care that does not attack the root cause, for example treatment as needed with pain-killers, oxygen, anti-nausea medication, etc., can also be used, and may be part of a treatment plan, or form the entire treatment plan itself. The second answer relating to why treat the underlying cancer if you can't cure it is more philosophical and each of us may have very different reactions to it. For myself, I tend to think about a number of different things including:

- Many serious and potentially life-shortening conditions are not curable, but we still treat them to maximize both our actual and potential quality and quantity of life—conditions such as HIV, diabetes, heart disease, asthma or COPD (chronic obstructive pulmonary disease). Drawing analogies between cancer and other serious life changing diseases such as HIV, severe heart disease or severe COPD probably seems pretty reasonable. However, for some subtypes of cancer, even the analogies with asthma and diabetes may become achievable goals within the next few years.

- In the worst case scenario—if the disease was going to end my life in a relatively short space of time—if the treatment could increase my chances of getting to a specific goal, an event I wanted to see or participate in on a specific date, like a wedding, Christmas or a family gathering, or just to give me time to set my affairs in order, I would consider it.

The treatments for most advanced cancers are not cures but attempts to control the disease. Even if control can be achieved, it does not last forever. Instead, multiple different treatments, called the first, second, third, etc., 'line' of treatment are usually employed. Each may produce or not produce control, and the extent and duration of the disease control produced by each one can vary enormously.

Consequently, treatment for advanced cancer is characterized by a recurring three-way decision point that, as the patient, you find yourself coming back to at the consideration of each new line of therapy: (1) Just treat the symptoms, (2) Treat the symptoms and have standard anti-cancer therapy, or (3) Treat the symptoms and have anti-cancer therapy within a clinical trial (Figure 1). Which of the three pathways is most attractive to you or most appropriate will vary. Each time it will depend on your own fitness, your own state-of-mind and the details of the side-effects, inconvenience and chances of success from the anti-cancer treatments that are available at that particular line of therapy/point in time.

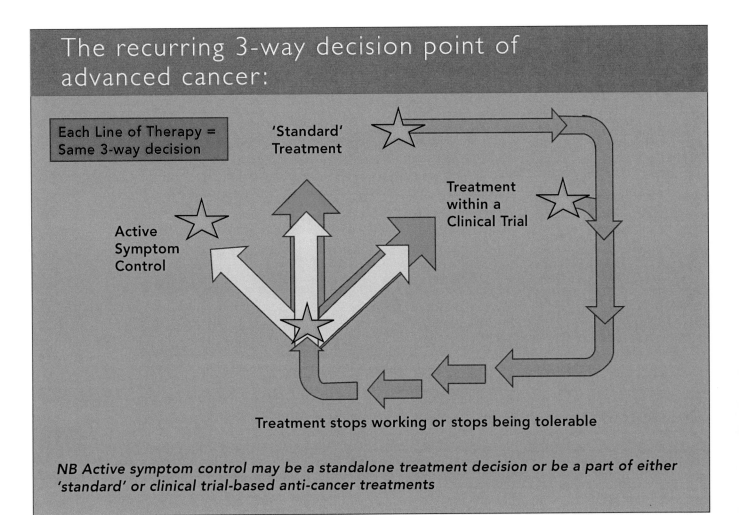

The recurring 3-way decision point of advanced cancer:

Each Line of Therapy = Same 3-way decision

'Standard' Treatment

Treatment within a Clinical Trial

Active Symptom Control

Treatment stops working or stops being tolerable

NB Active symptom control may be a standalone treatment decision or be a part of either 'standard' or clinical trial-based anti-cancer treatments

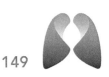

## 3) Clinical Trials—Overview:

Assume for a moment that you are not a participant in a trial, but just a consumer of the data coming out of them. Clinical trials establish for all of us a means to determine the best treatment for a specific condition, in a specific indication, at any particular point in time—for this cancer or that cancer; in the early, locally advanced or metastatic setting; in the metastatic setting in the first, second, third line of therapy, etc. This is established based on good evidence and free from prejudice, through a highly regulated, multi-step process. It aims to put decision-making on an objective level, above that of the whims of those who just want to sell us something, or of those who just have a gut feeling that something is right or wrong for us.

BUT…in the middle of dealing with a diagnosis of cancer, when your doctor brings up the idea of a clinical trial that you yourself might be involved in, it can be a source of enormous stress:

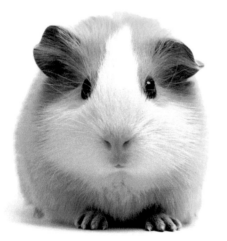

- *I don't understand this—it's too much to think about.*
- *What if it's a dumb idea, how can I tell?*
- *I don't want my decision to upset my doctor/my family*
- *I don't want to be a guinea pig.*
- *What if I get a placebo (dummy treatments)?*
- *What about the side effects?*
- *Who is paying for this?*

# GUINEA PIG?

So let's look into clinical trials in more detail— what they are, and what to look out for.

## 4) Where do clinical trials fit in?

Most clinical trials for cancer are in the advanced disease setting, fitting in as a treatment choice at a particular line of therapy. Clinical trials in early stage and locally advanced disease also exist, but are rarer and are usually only large phase III studies (see below). This is because cure is considered a more realistic possibility in these settings, so any new drug or other treatment change has to have a large amount of evidence behind it before anyone usually considers messing with a potentially curative standard approach.

Although there can be trials of anything—from a diagnostic test, to surgery, to radiotherapy, to symptomatic care, to counseling—most anti-cancer clinical trials involve the development and integration of new drugs. Therefore, for simplicities sake, from here on we will only illustrate this article with reference to anti-cancer **drug** trials. A clinical drug trial can be:

- *A new treatment on its own.*
- *A new treatment added into a standard treatment.*
- *A new treatment on its own, or added into standard treatment,* **compared to** *standard treatment alone (randomized study).*

Randomized studies may be open-label—where you know which of the available treatments that are being compared you are getting—or it may be 'blinded.' A 'blinded' study is one in which the study is 'placebo-controlled'—whereby you may be getting a dummy treatment or the new treatment, either on its own or added into standard therapy —but you, and probably your doctor too, won't know which of the two you are getting (although, code numbers will reveal it at a later date to the organizers of the study). It is also important to note that sometimes, where something is being compared to a 'standard treatment,' the standard may, in fact, be active symptom control alone, i.e. there is no standard anti-cancer treatment for that disease in that particular setting.

## 5) Do I qualify for a clinical trial?

Generally speaking, there is no point even looking at a trial that you do not qualify for. Most trials are asking specific questions and do not have too much room to bend their particular rules of eligibility. Therefore your doctor should have identified you as at least potentially eligible before mentioning any specific trial to you, so that neither of you waste time and energy thinking about something that this is never really going to be an option. Each trial has specific inclusion and exclusion criteria associated with it that your doctor can look up in advance to see if you are likely to be eligible. While sometimes eligibility or ineligibility is easy to determine straight away—for example, if you have colon cancer you won't qualify for a study designed only for those with breast cancer, or if you have early stage disease you won't qualify for a study designed for advanced stage disease, etc. Other issues on which people fail to qualify for clinical trials may not be apparent until more information or more test results about you become available. The three most common reasons that cause people with cancer to fail to qualify for clinical trials are inappropriate line of therapy, inadequate fitness for participation, and, less frequently, inappropriate insurance coverage. Dealing with each in turn:

**5a) Line of therapy:** A line of therapy is a full course of treatment, usually involving multiple different repeated exposures (cycles), with a specific drug or combination of drugs for advanced cancer. Each new drug or set of drugs that is tried to get your cancer under control is a line of therapy and is numbered sequentially—first line, second line, third line, etc. Using non-small cell lung cancer as the example again, a combination of carboplatin and paclitaxel for six cycles would be a common first line treatment (the two drugs being counted together as the first line regimen). Then this might be followed by, say, multiple cycles of pemetrexed started when the cancer begins to grow again (second line treatment), which might then be followed by tablets Erlotinib (Tarceva) at the point when the pemetrexed stops keeping the cancer under control (third line treatment). For different cancers the specific drugs and number of cycles will vary, but the principles of naming each new regimen of drugs used to try to get the cancer under control as sequentially numbered 'lines of therapy' ('lines of defense') remains the same. Of note, the same drug can be part of different lines of therapy in different individuals. For example, maybe Mr. Smith gets pemetrexed with carboplatin as part of his first-line treatment, instead of the paclitaxel, whereas Mr. Jones gets pemetrexed **after** his carboplatin and paclitaxel combination, in which case the pemetrexed would be his second line treatment.

Not all clinical trials are written in the same way, but most Phase II and III studies are constrained to only look at a particular line of therapy, i.e. you may be eligible if you have had two previous different treatments but not three, or one but not two, etc. Phase I studies (see below) are a notable exception to this and are often open to people regardless of the number of lines of therapy they have had. Areas of controversy that vary between studies include (a) whether **any** drug exposure counts—even if the treatment is then abandoned early because of side effects or allergic reactions—or whether it has to be shown to not be working on the cancer by scans showing that the cancer is growing despite the treatment, (b) whether any treatment given around the time of surgery (adjuvant or neo-adjuvant treatment) for early stage disease counts if you later relapse with more advanced stage disease, and (c) whether all drugs count the same or whether, for example, only chemotherapies are counted and so-called 'targeted therapies,' such as Erlotinib (Tarceva), are somehow "counted" differently. The reasoning behind this last point is that when cancers become resistant to one type of chemotherapy there can be a spill-over effect such that they also become partially resistant to other chemotherapies (this is why line of therapy is perceived to be important to level the playing field for any new drug in a particular setting). However, 'cross-resistance' to chemotherapies may not affect drugs that work very differently, such as highly targeted therapies where the presence or absence of a specific molecular factor may be a much more important determinant of the drug's activity or inactivity, and, as such, line of therapy in relation to prior chemotherapies may be a much less important variable affecting activity for these types of drugs.

**5b) Fitness for participation:** In some ways all participants in clinical trials are acting like test pilots—putting a new drug or combination of drugs through its paces, and figuring out what they do well, in the form of anti-cancer activity, and what they don't do well, in the form of side-effects or treatment-related 'toxicity.' As the number of people who have tried out a new drug will vary over time, just as in the real world of test pilots, it makes sense to only allow your best and fittest test pilots to try out the most experimental of your airplanes. In the world of clinical trials this means setting some benchmarks of fitness that patients need to achieve in order to be eligible for particular studies for safety reasons to allow them a good chance of being able to cope with unexpected severe or serious side effects should they occur. Fitness requirements are usually highest for Phase I studies and lowest for Phase III studies, as knowledge and confidence relating to the new drug increases over time. 'Fitness' doesn't necessarily mean physical fitness—although a patient's general 'performance status' is one thing that is considered—instead it often means simply that your kidneys and liver are working fine, or that you are not on medications with a strong potential to interact with the study drug, or that you do not have particular risk factors putting you at increased risk of side effects from the drug, such as a recent heart attack or stroke. Increasingly, 'fitness' for some of the newest targeted drugs may also mean having a test performed on the original biopsy of your cancer that may be stored away in a lab somewhere, in order to see if your cancer expresses a marker that makes it more likely that you will respond to the new drug or at least reduce the chances that you will be resistant to it— these molecular tests are sometimes called 'predictive biomarkers.' Perhaps the most frustrating thing about the fitness hurdles that an individual may have to clear in order to be eligible for a particular clinical study is that some of them are outside the control of the individual. You can be made ineligible on the basis of a simple blood test, even though you may feel like superman or superwoman at the time. While occasionally, at least from a Clinical Trialist's perspective, some studies are written too cautiously, in general, most of these rules are put there with the best intentions of protecting the

patient from excessive risks associated with their entry into a particular study.

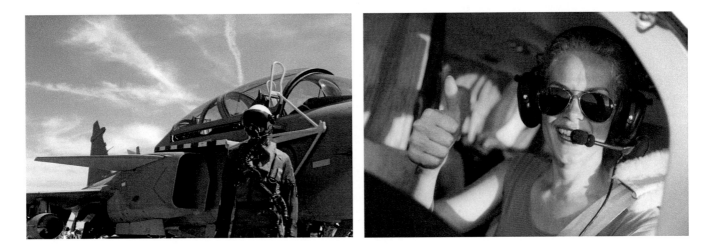

**5c) Insurance coverage:** There are many different trials, different sponsors of trials and different insurance programs. However, in general, the payment of costs associated with most clinical trials tends to follow the same basic principles. Firstly, if the trial includes elements of standard care—for example, standard chemotherapy drugs in addition to, or as an alternative to, any experimental drugs, routine visits to the doctor or routine scans to assess whether the treatment is working—these will be billed to your insurance. If you normally have co-pays for these things then that will not change. For 'extra' things associated with the study—research blood tests or research scans, any experimental drugs, even any extra visits to the clinic—usually these are not billed to your insurance but are absorbed by the sponsor of the study (usually either a pharmaceutical company or an academic individual or institution with a grant from the government or another organization that funds research, such as certain charities). Some insurance programs will not cover any aspects of clinical trials. However, this is the exception rather than the rule. If it happens, sometimes your doctor can explain matters to your insurance company, sometimes they can't. Since we are talking about costs, one thing that it is important to ask is if you need emergency care because of something directly related to the study—from an extra visit to your doctor to address side effects, to admission to hospital because of the severity of these side effects—would this care be perceived as standard, or as study-specific costs. The other thing to clarify is that, if you are receiving benefit from continued use of the study drug, you will still to be able to receive the drug for free, even if it ultimately gets licensed and other people starting on it are then being billed for it.

## 6) What does being in a trial involve?

Being in a clinical trial involves different things at different stages. At the beginning it involves taking on board some additional stresses—will you pass the screening tests? There are usually more unknowns about the side effects and efficacy of the treatment than with standard treatment—do these risks seem acceptable in return for the potential benefits of being in the study? Are any extra visits or tests acceptable to you in terms of the additional time commitment they involve?

To help you in making these decisions, all clinical trials involve the potential participant being shown a detailed 'consent form' that outlines what is known about the experimental treatment and any alternative treatments. It also describes what being in the study might involve and opportunity to read the consent form and to ask any questions you may have before deciding on whether this is something you want to take further.

The concept of 'informed consent,' i.e. giving you as much information in advance to help you decide about whether you give your consent to be screened for a given trial or not, is at the heart of all modern clinical trials. The amount of information available on any particular new drug will vary depending on whether the study is a Phase I, II or III study. The later the stage, the more is known about the drug. It doesn't necessarily mean the drug is any better or worse—just that the number of 'knowns' and 'unknowns' about it change as time goes by and more people are treated with it.

The other core concept is that you can withdraw consent at any time. The signing of a consent form doesn't force you into anything—you can always change your mind. The only consequence being that, if you do withdraw consent, you will then be withdrawn from the study and all or part of its associated experimental treatments. Most study teams try to be flexible— we all have to live in the real world and sometimes you can't make a particular appointment on a particular day—but in general there is an expected mutual agreement to try to abide by what the trial involves as much as possible. If you start to compromise the essence of the study too much, the investigator also has the right to withdraw you from the study, too.

Being in a study, after you have passed any screening tests, involves a mutual relationship of good two-way communication between you and the study staff (nurses, nurse practitioners, study coordinators (sometimes called CRAs—clinical research assistants, and physicians). It involves agreeing to report any side effects, any improvements, perhaps keeping track of whether you miss any doses of tablets, etc., and feeding these all back to the study team—just like a test pilot would frequently radio back to the control-tower about how a new airplane was handling.

# TEST PILOTS

157

**7) What are the potential advantages of being in a clinical trial?**

Broadly speaking, there are three main advantages to being on a study:

1.  The evolution of new knowledge that may help others know what is the best available treatment for their condition in the future.

2.  An individual on a study may get access to a better (more effective or less toxic) new treatment than is currently not available outside of a clinical study. However, it is important to remember that a new treatment may NOT be better than what is already out there (otherwise we wouldn't need to do the trial to prove it). It is also important to remember that, if you are considering a randomized study (see below), you may end up getting the same standard treatment that you would get off-study and not getting the new treatment at all.

3.  Being in a clinical study involves forming a close relationship with a dedicated team of experts focused on your care that may bring many general health benefits—such as having a larger number of named individuals to contact for help or advice, or spotting and acting on other conditions, symptoms or side effects earlier than might happen with standard medical care. For this reason, I clearly recall one trial participant commenting that in her clinical trial she didn't feel at all like a guinea pig, but more like a prize poodle—with her own entourage of people fussing over her and making sure everything was just as good as it could possibly be.

# PRIZE POODLE

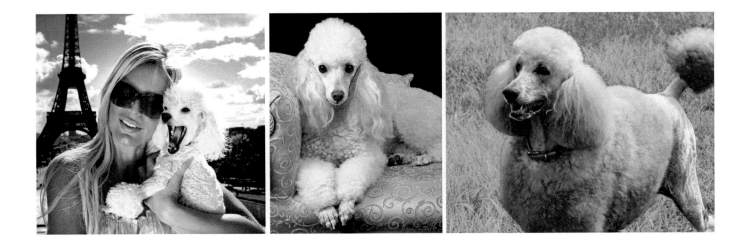

## 8) How do I know if a particular trial is a dumb idea or not?

Despite other reasons, most of us will still only be considering a trial for the express reason of getting access to something **new**. So how do we tell if new is better? When you're not a doctor or a molecular biologist, how do you tell if a trial is looking at something promising and that it's not just some crazy idea that could be wasting your time?

Firstly, we should be reassured that all clinical trials, in the USA and in most other developed countries, are very carefully regulated. Since the Nuremberg trials of the Nazis', international consensus on how clinical trials should be conducted has existed. International guidelines, for example, within something called the Declaration of Helsinki, are regularly updated and expected to be followed. For an individual trial, once the trial is written and before any patient can be entered onto the study, it has to be approved by a series of local committees—usually involving some kind of scientific review and some kind of ethical review to confirm that it makes sense and is in concordance with such international guidelines. If it involves a new drug, then it also has to be encompassed within an Investigational New Drug (IND) listing registered with the US Food and Drug Administration (FDA). So crazy ideas for clinical trials, in theory, shouldn't get anywhere near you.

However, it is still vitally important to ask your doctor two questions about any particular

***1. How much is known about this new treatment?***
***2. What are my options if I don't go on this study?***

More than almost anything else, the answers you get to these simple questions will help you to decide if a clinical trial in a particular setting is really the right thing for you to participate in or not. So let's deal with each in turn:

**8a) What is known about this treatment?—Phases I, II and III.**

Whether a study is labeled as a Phase I, Phase II or Phase III study generates a lot of debate. In reality it is not that big a deal. All the Phase of the study tells you is how much is known about the drug, and what being in the study might involve in terms of intensity of visits and chances of it being a randomized study—in and of itself it doesn't tell you whether a drug is better or worse than anything else. In the hands of an expert the right drug for you may be accessed through any Phase of clinical trials.

**i) Phase I studies:**

All drugs, when they are first given to humans, have to explore the correct dose to give —either on their own or in combination with other drugs. These dose-finding studies are called Phase I studies. Because they happen early on in the life of a new drug, there are more unknowns than in later Phase studies, and they are, by definition, the most experimental of studies. Phase I studies tend to be open to anyone with any type of advanced cancer at any line of therapy. Traditionally, they were for those individuals who had exhausted most, perhaps even all, standard treatments. However, in recent years, as specifically targeted drugs that may have particular promise in certain diseases have been developed, in some situations Phase I studies of new drugs, or new drugs in combination with established first-line treatments, may be considered much earlier on in the treatment journey of some individuals.

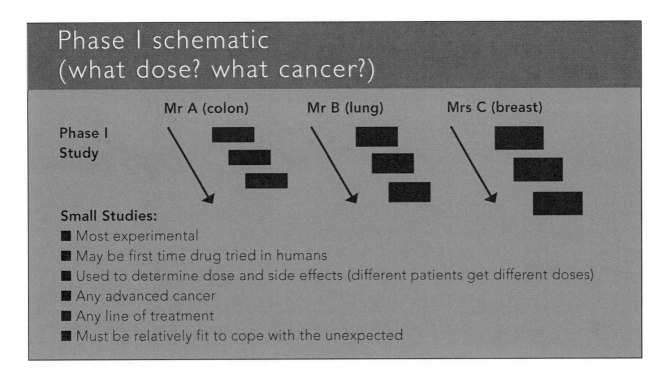

## Phase I schematic (what dose? what cancer?)

Mr A (colon)    Mr B (lung)    Mrs C (breast)

Phase I Study

**Small Studies:**
■ Most experimental
■ May be first time drug tried in humans
■ Used to determine dose and side effects (different patients get different doses)
■ Any advanced cancer
■ Any line of treatment
■ Must be relatively fit to cope with the unexpected

As Phase I studies are dose-finding studies, participants who enter the study when it first opens will get a lower dose of drug than participants who enter at a later time point. In general, the dose of the drug is increased with each new group of participants entering the study, with an individual tending to stick at the dose they started on. Some people worry whether, if they are in the first few dose levels, they will get effective doses of the drug. On the other hand, if you are in the last few dose levels, people worry about whether they will get too much in the way of side effects. There isn't a simple response to reassure participants as to these worries. However, it is important to note that some of the newest drugs can achieve efficacy at levels well below those that produce side effects. Also, to remember that side effects are very carefully monitored at all times during these studies, to try and ultimately choose a tolerable dose to take forward to other studies, not an intolerable one. Participants have to be fairly fit to enter Phase I studies in order to cope with the unexpected. Also, the number of study-specific visits and tests tend to be more than in any other Phase of clinical studies. In general, observations and tests are more intensive at the start of the study. Then, after about a month on study, they become much less frequent as it is clear at that point how well you are tolerating the treatment. For safety reasons, after a certain number of patients start at a particular dose there is usually an observation period (about 3 weeks) during which they are treated and when no one else can join the study, until it is clear how well that particular dose level is tolerated. All patients on all Phases of clinical studies should have routine scans or other assessments to confirm that their disease is being kept under control or is responding to treatment. If the drug is not working for you, or you cannot tolerate the drug, usually you will come off the study and return to the three-way decision point outlined above with regard to what you should do next.

## Phase I example (Mrs A)

- Advanced Sarcoma
- Exhausted standard chemotherapy
- Came to UCCC Phase I practice
- One of the first 50 people to try experimental drug
- Seen every week for the first month, now every few months
- Possible side effects: intermittent fatigue; previous area of radiotherapy became inflamed
- Activity: Slow progressive shrinkage of tumors, great disease control for almost 2 years now

## ii) Phase II Studies

Once a Phase I study is complete, the drug—at the doses determined as appropriate to take forward based on the results of the Phase I study—is then explored in a series of Phase II studies to get a good feel for its activity in different cancers at that dose. Of note, if you started on the Phase I study and the drug is still working for you, you stay in the Phase I study. It is the drug which expands to start a new study, not you. Within Phase II studies usually all patients receive the same dose of drug and, because more is known about the side effects and tolerability of the drug, the fitness requirements for entry tend to get more relaxed and the number of study-specific visits and tests also get less. However, at this point the manufacturer of the drug is starting to look for a specific license for the drug, so Phase II studies are usually restricted both by tumor type (there may be several parallel Phase II studies, each in a different tumor type) and by line of therapy (usually first, second or third line of therapy, but not beyond this).

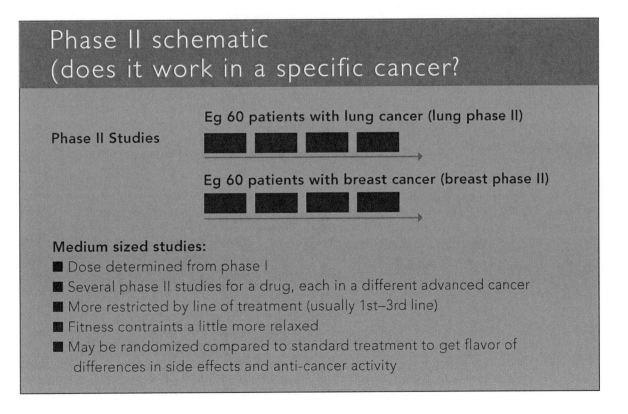

Phase II schematic
(does it work in a specific cancer?

**Phase II Studies**

**Eg 60 patients with lung cancer (lung phase II)**

**Eg 60 patients with breast cancer (breast phase II)**

**Medium sized studies:**
■ Dose determined from phase I
■ Several phase II studies for a drug, each in a different advanced cancer
■ More restricted by line of treatment (usually 1st–3rd line)
■ Fitness contraints a little more relaxed
■ May be randomized compared to standard treatment to get flavor of differences in side effects and anti-cancer activity

Phase II studies may be randomized (see below), comparing two different doses of the same drug or different treatment regimens, or to get a first look at the new treatment compared to some standard treatment. However, although randomization is becoming more common, most Phase II studies are still not randomized. Instead, most randomized studies are Phase III studies.

## Phase II example (Mrs B)

- Advanced lung cancer that had responded to one treatment but then grew again
- Phase II study looking at new tablet that looks promising in lung cancer (second line treatment)
- Dose determined from previous phase I study
- Side effects: rash and diarrhea
- Activity: Dramatic improvement in scans, came off oxygen, and good disease control for 2 years to date

### iii) Phase III Studies:

Once a drug has (a) its dose determined from a Phase I study and (b) some signal as to which tumor type it might work in from the Phase II studies, in order to get a license from the FDA, usually it has to be shown to be at least as good or better than what is already available for treating a particular cancer. This kind of large comparative study, almost always randomized against some current standard treatment, is called a Phase III study.

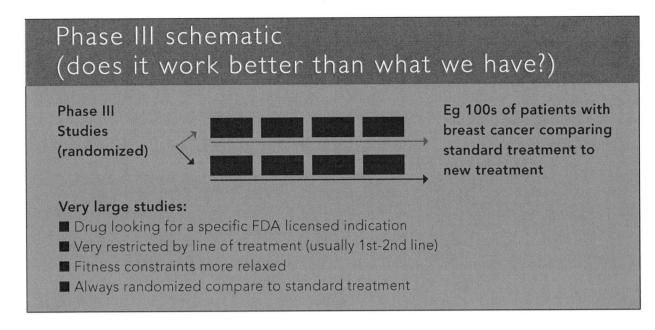

Phase III schematic
(does it work better than what we have?)

Phase III
Studies
(randomized)

Eg 100s of patients with breast cancer comparing standard treatment to new treatment

**Very large studies:**
■ Drug looking for a specific FDA licensed indication
■ Very restricted by line of treatment (usually 1st-2nd line)
■ Fitness constraints more relaxed
■ Always randomized compare to standard treatment

As this may be the final step before a drug is licensed, Phase III studies are the most restrictive in terms of tumor type and line of therapy. Although, as they are trying to develop something for use in the wider community and knowledge about the specific new drug will have increased from the time of the earlier studies, they may be less restrictive in terms of general fitness. Everyday pilots, in addition to the very Top Gun test pilots, may be eligible to participate.

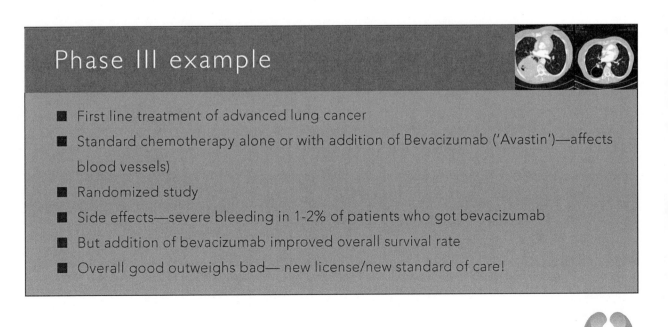

Phase III example

■ First line treatment of advanced lung cancer
■ Standard chemotherapy alone or with addition of Bevacizumab ('Avastin')—affects blood vessels)
■ Randomized study
■ Side effects—severe bleeding in 1-2% of patients who got bevacizumab
■ But addition of bevacizumab improved overall survival rate
■ Overall good outweighs bad— new license/new standard of care!

165

In general, if you are in the first or second line of treatment for advanced cancer, you will mostly be considering Phase II or Phase III studies. If you are at third line or beyond you will mostly only have Phase I studies open to you. However, as mentioned previously, the Phase of the study really only tells you how much is already known about the drug and the level of intensive investigation/extra visits/ extra tests and/or the chances of the study being a randomized study. It doesn't tell you if a drug will work or not and an expert physician may seek out the best drug for you in studies of any Phase. Being cared for in a center where the doctors have expert knowledge of your disease and a large palette of available studies to choose from in order to select the best drug for you at each line of treatment is therefore something to be strongly considered. If you have the means, the insurance, the fitness and/or the inclination to travel, then a large list of clinical trials— complete with a search engine to allow you to narrow down to your particular tumor type and line of therapy—can be found at **www.clinicaltrials.gov.** Your physician will **not** know every trial that is going on around the country, so it's perfectly acceptable to do some homework in your own time and ask your doctor's opinion on the different studies. However, unless there is a true breakthrough out there that has to be searched out and is only available within a clinical trial, most people do not travel too far for clinical trials—especially if the trial they were considering traveling for is a randomized trial with a chance that they could end up getting exactly the same as they would have got nearer to home.

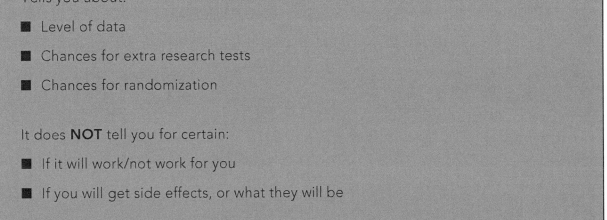

## Phase I-III—Does it matter?

Tells you about:

■ Level of data

■ Chances for extra research tests

■ Chances for randomization

It does **NOT** tell you for certain:

■ If it will work/not work for you

■ If you will get side effects, or what they will be

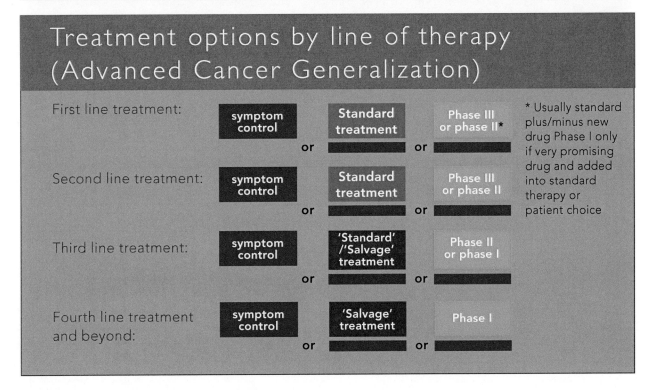

## Treatment options by line of therapy (Advanced Cancer Generalization)

| First line treatment: | symptom control | or | Standard treatment | or | Phase III or phase II* | * Usually standard plus/minus new drug Phase I only if very promising drug and added into standard therapy or patient choice |
| Second line treatment: | symptom control | or | Standard treatment | or | Phase III or phase II | |
| Third line treatment: | symptom control | or | 'Standard' /'Salvage' treatment | or | Phase II or phase I | |
| Fourth line treatment and beyond: | symptom control | or | 'Salvage' treatment | or | Phase I | |

In the Figure above, 'salvage' treatment usually means other kinds of 'traditional' chemotherapy that are available, but that may not be formally licensed in your particular cancer. Sometimes there is still a 'chink' in the cancer's armor that these different variants of traditional chemotherapy can exploit. However, sometimes cancers develop cross-resistance to many different chemotherapy drugs, such that increasing lines of traditional salvage chemotherapy start to manifest the law of 'diminishing returns.' My own opinion is that, sometime before you start exploring traditional drugs that are somehow 'left in the cupboard,' you should have at least explored your options for treatment within clinical trials, too. The drugs left in the cupboard will still be there for you to explore after considering clinical trials, but you may be excluded from some clinical trials if you've had too many different chemotherapies, or your fitness has slipped too much while you are working your way through these salvage treatments.

**8b) What are my options if I don't go into this study? If it's a randomized study, what might I be randomized to?**

Having got your head around what a clinical study is, what informed consent means, and whether you might qualify for a study, the single most important question to understand is what your treatment options are if you don't go on the study. In part, this is to help you finalize your thoughts on whether you want to enter the study —how many visits and tests would you have if you weren't on the study, is there a standard treatment that you would miss out on if you went on the study, etc. However, the most important reason to ask this question is if this is a randomized study. More than almost anything else, randomization—a computer tossing a coin and determining which of two or more different treatments you will end up getting—causes the most stress when an individual is trying to decide on whether to enter a clinical study or not. When it's a placebo—controlled study—i.e. you may be getting a dummy treatment instead of the real treatment—this just increases the stress levels even more.

So why do studies bother with randomization? The short answer is it's the only way to be certain if a new treatment is really better or not. People talk about the 'placebo effect,' when our minds make us think we're feeling better (or sometimes worse) after taking a particular treatment, even when it's just a sugar tablet. So if you want to really prove to the FDA that your drug actually works, you have to eventually compare it to something in a head-to-head, pepsi-cola versus coca-cola kind of challenge. Placebos (which can be dummy tablets or dummy injections) are sometimes used to distinguish drug effects from the side effects of just taking any kind of tablet or injection, and to minimize the risks of people withdrawing consent from a randomized study if they don't end up randomized to the arm they want. Although the possibilities of randomization and of placebos can be stressful things, they do have their roles to play in helping us all out in terms of truly determining the next best treatment. To deal with these stresses though, consider the following checklist to ask your doctor about any study:

1.      Is this a randomized study? If it is, you have to be told what the possible treatments are and your numerical chances of being allocated to each treatment 'arm.'

2.      If it is a randomized study, is there a placebo arm? If there is, as part of informed consent you have to be told this in advance, and your numerical chances of getting the placebo (e.g. 50:50).

3.      If there is a placebo—is it the whole treatment (i.e. could you be getting just symptom control) or does everyone get some kind of anti-cancer treatment and the placebo or study drug is then just added in on top? Either is possible, mostly depending on whether there is a perceived standard that everyone should be getting at that line of treatment.

4.      If there is a placebo arm to the study and the drug doesn't work—will your doctor be able to find out (quickly) if you did get the placebo and offer you the other treatment? This is called 'unblinding' and 'crossing over.' Its availability varies but is a nice aspect of a study if it's there—a second chance.

5.      If there is no placebo, just a comparison of two different treatments—pepsi-cola versus coca-cola—it is VERY important to clarify if the 'standard' treatment arm is the same standard that you would be offered if you weren't on the study.

169

# I cannot emphasize this last point enough.

On a simple level, let's say there are normally two different standard chemotherapies, both equally effective at treating your cancer, but one is given half as often as the other (less visits) but it also makes your hair fall out, whereas the other one doesn't. If you weren't in the study, you would have a choice between the pros and cons of these two treatments. Within a randomized study of new drug X added into standard chemotherapy, it is likely that only one of these standard chemotherapy regimens will have been chosen. In the study, you may be randomized to standard chemo (the one that is given less frequently, but that makes your hair fall out) or to the same standard chemotherapy plus new drug X. Here, by knowing what your options 'off-study' are, you can make the choice of whether you want to go in the study to potentially have the benefits of the new drug and/or the general benefits of being in a study, but limit your choice of the standard chemotherapy you receive to only the one that makes you lose your hair (which may or may not be a big deal to you—but, either way, it should be part of your informed decision-making process).

On a more complex and more serious level, knowing what your options off study are is incredibly important because randomized studies can sometimes get out of date while they are still going on. Let me explain what I mean by this. Let's say the standard treatment is chemotherapy with drugs A and B combined, and you are being offered a randomized Phase III study of A plus B compared to A plus B plus X (where X is a new drug). Phase III studies require hundreds, sometimes thousands, of patients to be recruited and their results analyzed to determine whether the addition of X (or its equivalent) is worthwhile in terms of its extra side effects and any extra anti-cancer efficacy. If you look at **www.clinicaltrials.gov** or surf the Internet at all looking for anticancer trials you will see that there are many different trials all going on at the same time. So what happens if, over night, A plus B is no longer the appropriate standard?

What if someone finds out either that A plus B is less safe for people like you, or that C plus D is actually a better treatment than A plus B for your particular kind of cancer? Your planned randomized study may still be going on; however, the new information is something that you probably would want to know to weigh up whether the chances of getting access to new drug X with A plus B, still outweighs the new information relating to C plus D as the new standard treatment for your disease. Therefore, the single most important thing to do is:

# Ask your doctor: "If I don't go into this study, what would you treat me with?"

Only when you have asked this question (and are happy with the answer!) can you truly weigh up the pros and cons of being entered into a randomized clinical study.

### 9) What if the 'best' treatment is redefined while I am on a study—can I, or should I, change treatment?

This is a tough one to answer. It is imagining a situation in which you have started on a treatment plan (which may, or may not, be part of a study) and suddenly there is a breakthrough announced that there is another treatment, or something added into the kind of treatment you are already on, that may be better than your current treatment plan. I think here I would discuss it with your doctor and, if it's safe and you are not on a trial, ask about whether you can 'upgrade' to the new standard. If you are on a clinical trial, you probably have less flexibility as the study will probably not update that quickly. Instead you have to decide if the advance could make enough of a difference that you should consider withdrawing from the study to change to this new standard. The things to think about here are firstly, how much longer you may have to go on the study

171

treatment, particularly, if it is only for a defined number of cycles. If you only have one more cycle to go there is probably no point jumping ship at this point. Secondly, to recognize that if in the clinical trial you are not just on the original standard treatment, but on the standard plus something else, you won't know if the 'new standard' is, in fact, better than the **even** 'newer' regimen that you are being treated with. If you are on a randomized study then you need to ask if you are definitely getting the new treatment or not. If you and your doctor don't know (i.e. if it is a 'blinded' placebo-controlled study) you would have to weigh up the chances that you are actually receiving the study treatment against the pros and cons of coming off the study to switch to the new standard that has just been defined. In reality, these situations don't come up very often and in the past the 'new' standards, at least in my experience, have **not** been such big breakthroughs. Consequently, I usually don't recommend changing horses mid-stream. However, it's important to have the discussion and to make the decision you feel most comfortable with. If you've already completed the treatment, changes to what that standard **was** will cause you some stress, but there's not much you can do. While it may be appropriate for you to try the new treatment in a later line of therapy, you cannot change what has already happened.

## 10) If I go on a study how long am I on the study for?

In general you would stay being treated within a study until one of the following occurred:

1.  The drug was proven to not be working for you (usually on the basis of some unfavorable change in your disease, for example demonstrating tumor growth on your scans).

2.    The side effects of the drug meant that it wasn't tolerable for you. Sometimes the dose of the study drug can be reduced and retried at the lower dose, but after a couple of dose reductions, if you're still having problems most people would have to walk away from a drug that they just couldn't take.

3.    You have completed a fixed number of cycles of treatment predefined by the study—for example 4 to 6 cycles of many traditional chemotherapies is about all that most people can tolerate and about all the good that can be done by the chemotherapy is completed within that time. However, this is not the case for some of the newer treatments, which are both better tolerated and work in a very different way from traditional chemotherapy. For example, defining a fixed number of cycles would be very unusual for most of the latest, so called targeted agents.

4.    You change your mind and withdraw your consent.

However, even if you are not being treated, most studies will still be collecting some information on you. For example, the time it takes for your cancer to start to grow again, whether your cancer has returned or not, or simply that you're still alive and kicking. Laboratory tests on blood samples or tumor specimens that you may have given permission for may also be ongoing for years after you have completed treatment in order to determine, in retrospect, what the people who did well or who did badly had in common on a molecular level.

## Clinical Trials Decision Guide

- ■ Do I qualify?

- ■ Will my insurance cover the standards of care?

- ■ What are my options if I don't go in this study?

- ■ What is known about the side effects?

- ■ What has been seen so far to make you think this may or may not work?

- ■ How many extra visits/tests are involved?

(answers to most of these questions will vary with Phase I-III)

## Randomized Study Decision Guide

- ■ Is this a randomized study? **Will I definitely get the new treatment?**

- ■ If this **is** a randomized study, will I know which treatment I am getting? **Is there a placebo?**

- ■ If this **is** a randomized study and I get the standard treatment, is this any different from what you would give me if I wasn't in the study?

**VERY IMPORTANT!**

**11) In summary:**

Clinical trials are essential for progress, to help each of us know the best treatment for different diseases at any given point in time. Sometimes, the information we generate from being involved in clinical trials helps others. Sometimes, by being involved in the trial ourselves, there are general benefits from the more intensive care received. Sometimes, there are specific benefits if the trial involves access to a new treatment that actually is better. However, it is important to realize that new is not always better (otherwise we wouldn't need to do the trials). Also, to know that, in randomized trials, you may not automatically get the new treatment, or know if you are getting it or not.

Deciding whether you enter a trial can be a stressful task and the best thing to do is to ask lots of questions, seek opinions from friends, relatives or other professionals and understand the principles of informed consent—**you should never feel like a guinea pig —guinea pigs do not get a choice—you always do—and you can change your mind.**

Ideally, as there are always some unknowns associated with being in a clinical trial involving any new treatment—you should be fit enough to cope with some level of unexpected side effects, just in case you are the one person in which they do occur. Being in a trial means forming a close working relationship with the doctors and other staff associated with the study—good communication about what the study involves and how you are doing on the study—just like a test pilot's relationship with the control tower. Sometimes, being in a trial, even if you don't get one or other treatment, is beneficial in itself just because of the close relationship you form with your medical team—becoming one of the 'Prize Poodles' described in the title.

Entry into a trial is sometimes the right thing to do and sometimes not—and that may change over time—in part with the specifics of the trial, the current alternatives available and where you are in your own treatment journey. However, it is often something to at least consider discussing with an expert every time you find yourself at the recurring 3-way treatment decision point described earlier.

Without the test pilots and prize poodles (and hopefully not too many guinea pigs) who have gone before, we would still be listening to snake oil salesmen on the back of wagons. Within the last decade, I have already seen amazing things start to happen in our fight against many different types of cancer—progress that will increase as we all work towards the same goal: doctors, scientists, drug companies, study teams, test pilots and prize poodles all pulling together to make cancer a footnote not a headline in people's lives in the future.

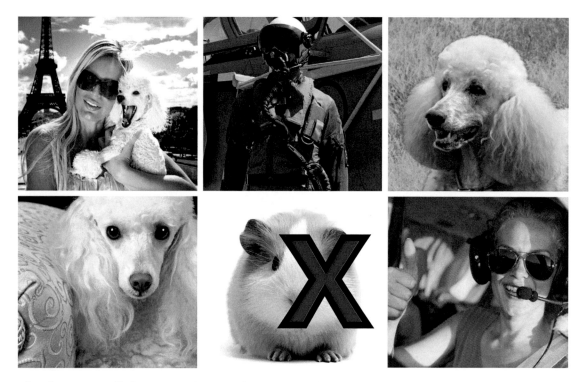

Thank you to all the Test Pilots and Prize Poodles who continue to help define (and redefine) the state-of-the-art in cancer care each and every year.

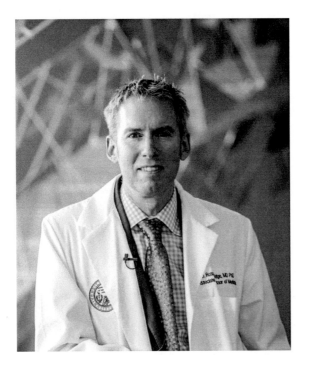

**About the Author:**

D. Ross Camidge qualified in Medicine from Oxford University in the UK, with a PhD in Molecular Biology from Cambridge University. He trained in both Medical Oncology and Clinical Pharmacology and is an expert in the development of new anti-cancer drugs. He joined the University of Colorado in 2005, initially as a Visiting Professor and then as full-time Faculty from October 2007. He is the Director of the Thoracic Oncology Clinical and Clinical Research Programs, as well as being a specialist  Attending Physician within the Developmental Therapeutics Program, at the University of Colorado Cancer Center.

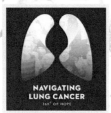

BRING HOPE HOME

**EVERY THIRD**

TUESDAY

# JOIN US! LIVE!

Whether you join us in the Living Room live or attend remotely through Ustream on your computer, you will be informed about living with lung cancer.

**WHO:** Lung Cancer Living Room Support Group

**WHEN:** Third Tuesday/monthly (5:30-7:30 PST)

**WHERE:** ALCF Living Room, 1100 Industrial Road, #1, San Carlos, California 94070

Or, from your living room: www.ustream.com and select **Lung Cancer Living Room Support Group Channel**

**WHAT:** Guest speakers, drinks and appetizers

**INFO:** Michele Zeh—Manager of Patient Services & Programs  michele@lungcancerfoundation.org

*Partners*

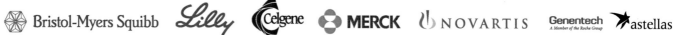
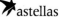

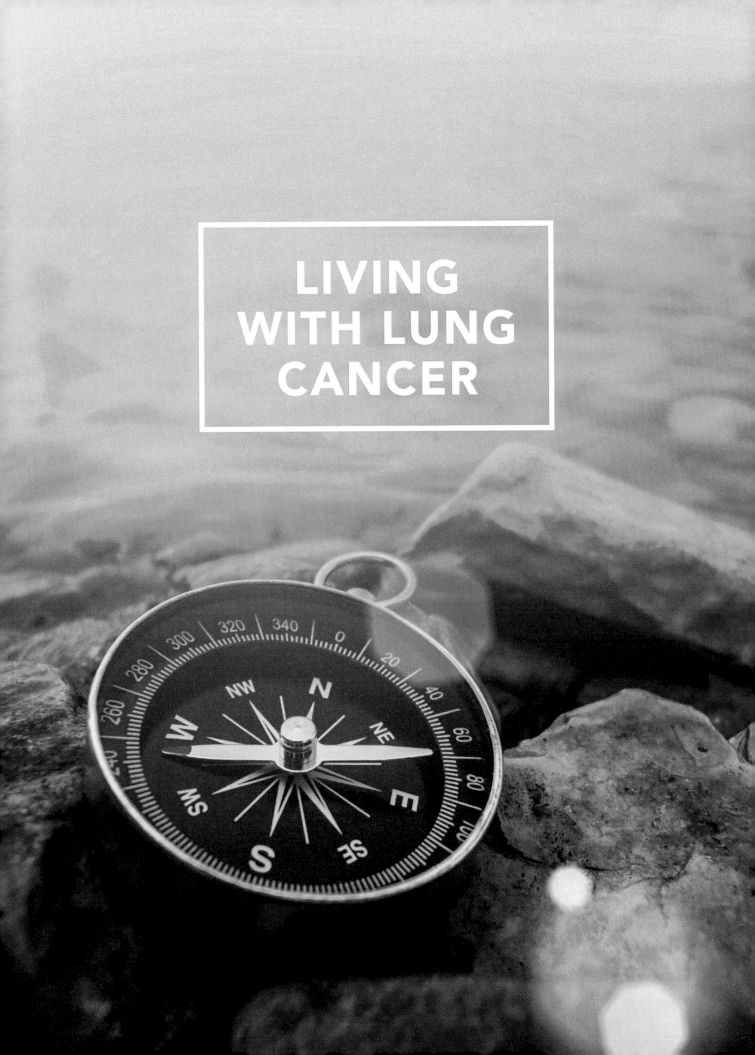

# LIVING WITH LUNG CANCER

*When you are overwhelmed or don't know where to turn, the Lung Cancer Foundation becomes a 'home' — a safe haven of caring people who will share their amazing knowledge and give you the courage and strength (along with faith in God) to face the journey knowing you are making the best possible choices for YOU."*

—Janice Lalley, survivor

# LIVING WITH LUNG CANCER

When you are diagnosed with lung cancer and start receiving treatments, you begin to realize the many changes that are happening in your life. As your health status and treatment plans change, the care you receive will also change. During these periods of change, you may have problems moving from one phase into the next. Your healthcare team should help you move between phases by working with you to create a Transitional Care Plan.

**Transitional Care Planning**

Transitional Care Planning will help you find a healthy balance between your disease and the rest of your life. While you have treatments, doctor's appointments, and days when you are not feeling your best, your family, finances, and job situation will continue to move on. You may become depressed or anxious about these issues that you just simply cannot manage right now. Transitional Care Planning can help you identify and manage these problems to minimize the impact on your treatment and healing process. Your healthcare team will help educate and support you and your family by providing support and providing referrals to resources that you may need during your care.

As your lung cancer gets better or worse, your treatment goals will change. During active treatment, you may be receiving chemotherapy, radiation, surgery, some combination therapy, or a new, experimental treatment. You will also be receiving supportive care to treat symptoms of the lung cancer and side effects from your treatments. Palliative therapy will be given to improve the quality of your life at any time in your cancer journey or to make you comfortable at the end of your life. Because each of these types of care are different, your Transitional Care Plan can help you and your family adjust by helping with the day-to-day issues, medical problems and emotional issues that will arise in each phase. And because you are a unique person, your Transitional Care

Plan will also be unique. Your healthcare team will do many assessments to determine what care is needed to make the changes you experience go smoothly.

## Transitional Care Planning Assessments

Some kind of assessment will be done at every contact with your healthcare team. Your oncologist will examine you, the nurse will ask about side effects, general health status, appetite, and any issues you may be having in your life. The social worker and/or financial counselor will help you with any issues you might be having in your employment or financial life. As your treatments change, your team will help to identify any new needs or stresses you or your family might have. Specifically, your healthcare team will do physical, care setting, support system, spiritual and mental health, and legal assessments. These assessments may not be done at every visit, but will certainly be done when there are changes in your health status or treatment plan.

### Physical Assessment

Throughout your treatment, but especially when you are diagnosed with lung cancer, when you are receiving treatments, or when there is a change in your treatment, you will receive regular physical assessments by various members of your healthcare team. In general, your doctors and nurses will be primarily responsible for your physical assessment. In addition to asking you questions about your symptoms and quality of life, the healthcare team will usually do a hands-on exam.

This exam might include:

- Measurement of your temperature, pulse, respiratory rate, weight and blood pressure
- General examination to look for signs of infection
- Listening to your heart and lungs
- Feeling your armpits, neck, groin and other areas of your body to check for swollen lymph nodes

- Drawing blood
- Doing x-rays or other radiological procedures
- Doing pulmonary (lung) tests to determine how your lungs are functioning

## Care Setting Assessment

During your treatments, you may receive treatment in many different care settings. Some of your care may occur in the hospital, but you may also receive care in an outpatient cancer center, home, a nursing home or a rehabilitation center. As your care moves from one setting to another, your healthcare team will help you plan for this change in care setting. New team members may become involved in your care; this will depend on the type of care you need at any given point in your cancer journey.

As you move from one care setting to another, your team will assess your needs and the physical arrangements in the new setting. If the team determines that you need medical equipment or assistive devices to help you move around, they will help you find those services.

## Support Systems Assessment

Your healthcare team will do a full assessment of your support systems—those people and groups around you who are willing to help you during your illness. This assessment will also include a review of those people for whom you might be responsible. If you have young children or elderly parents that you care for, your team will help you determine how roles and relationships might change during your treatments.

It is sometimes very hard to ask for help. However, this is one time when you will need people around you who care about you and are willing to help. We know that your loved ones and friends will feel honored when you ask them to help you during this journey. At the same time, you might find that you have many friends who want to help – and you may want one person to act as the gatekeeper. Your gatekeeper can be responsible for taking phone calls, answering emails, helping schedule visits and setting up a schedule for your friends who want to be involved with you during your treatment.

What things can your support team do for you? Of course, you are the one who is in control of the help you need, but your loved ones can help with specific tasks when you just don't feel up to doing daily chores. Duties that you might consider sharing with your team include things such as:

- Cooking meals for you and your family. Meals that can be frozen and defrosted for use at any time are particularly good.
- Babysitting. If you have young children, your friends with children may be very willing to take yours for a "play date." This may be useful when you are having treatments and have to be out of the house for several hours.
- Driving you to appointments. Many of the treatments you might receive can make you tired; having someone drive you to and from appointments will be critical. There may be other options available for transportation to and from appointments:
  – American Cancer Society's Road to Recovery: to find out if Road to Recovery is available in your area visit their website at
  http://www.cancer.org/Treatment/SupportProgramsServices/road-to-recovery
  or call 1-800-227-2345.
  –Cancer Care: provides free, professional support for anyone affected by cancer. To learn more about their programs visit. www.cancercare.org
  or call 1-800-813-HOPE (4673).

–Speak with your social worker. They may be able to direct you to a local transportation program.

–Local religious organizations may have people who would be happy to help you with transportation.

- Light housekeeping. Again, treatments are likely to make you feel tired. A friend will likely be thrilled if you ask for help with vacuuming or light dusting. If you need additional help with housekeeping activities, contact Cleaning For A Reason – the non-profit organization that connects maid services with women enduring cancer treatments. To learn more call 1-877-337-3348 or visit www.cleaningforareason.org.

- Lodging while a loved one is receiving treatment away from home. If you have to travel and stay overnight for your treatments, you and your family may need a place to stay. Often, your personal support system may have a place for you to stay. If not, there may be other resources available to you:

  –American Cancer Society's Hope Lodge: For more information on Hope Lodge visit their website at http://www.cancer.org/Treatment/SupportProgramsServices/HopeLodge/index

  –Joe's House, A Lodging Guide for Cancer Patients http://www.joeshouse.org/ or call 1-877-563-7468.

  –Ask your healthcare team if they know of discounted housing for out of town patients.

- Talking! You will probably want to talk to people throughout your treatment. Some of your support team will feel comfortable listening to you talk about your lung cancer; others will be great to sit and gossip with you. Both of these groups are important to you.

Anything else where you just need a friend to be with you. Remember, that your loved ones are likely to feel helpless, but they really want to help you. They will be honored that you asked them to help.

## Spiritual and Mental Health Assessment

When you receive a diagnosis of lung cancer, you will very likely experience a broad range of emotions. It is very likely that that your first reaction may be one of disbelief and denial – "There has to be a mistake. I can't have lung cancer." As you begin to accept that the diagnosis is real, you may feel angry – "This isn't fair. What did I do to deserve this?" It is also very common to get depressed and have feelings of hopelessness during your treatment. This is particularly true when you are not feeling well and find that you cannot do those things you can usually do. Throughout your treatment, you may very well be scared. This fear may be related to the diagnosis itself, the treatments you are going through, or simply the fear of the unknown. All of these reactions are normal.

During a spiritual or mental health assessment, your healthcare team will ask you questions about how you and your family feel about your treatments and treatment plan. They may ask you about what things are most important to you since those things will affect your plan. The team may ask questions about how you and your family usually deal with stress. Are there things you have done in the past that you can use during this time? Are there other stressors in the home that will interfere with treatment and your ability to concentrate on healing?

You may look to your church, religion or spiritual beliefs to help you cope with your diagnosis and treatments. There are studies that show that spirituality may help you adjust to your diagnosis and treatments in a way that will help you cope with the new stressors in your life. Your spirituality may be expressed as an organized religion, yoga, the arts, or any other outlet that allows you express your feelings about life. If you are a member of a religious or spiritual community or church, the other members of the community can be an excellent source of support to you and to your family.

The diagnosis of lung cancer has a profound effect on you, but it also has a huge impact on your loved ones. There are many support groups available to you and your family and friends. The ALCF Lung Cancer Living Room® is a monthly online support group that welcomes patients, families and friends. Our hope is that during these monthly meetings, we can share stories, talk about problems you are having, share ideas and practices that have helped, raise awareness of lung cancer, and offer any kind of support to patients, survivors and families. There are many other support groups. To find these groups, search "lung cancer support groups" online. Your local treatment center or hospital may also have a support group. Your social worker or case manager should be able to give you contact information for those groups.

Consider visiting the ALCF Lung Cancer Living Room® for support before, during and after treatment. This support group meets in person and online every third Tuesday of every month. Visit http://www.ustream.tv/channel/the-lung-cancer-living-room-support-group or email Hope@lungcancerfoundation.org or call us at 1-650-598-2857 for more information.

As you progress through treatment, dealing with stress and depression will be critical. If you find yourself having problems coping, ask your oncologist for a referral to a mental health professional. Depending on the kind of help you need, your doctor may refer you to one of a number of different professionals: psychiatrists, psychologists and psychiatric clinical nurse specialist. A psychiatrist is a medical doctor who provides counseling, medication and other treatments for mental and emotional disorders. A clinical psychologist is a professional with advanced training in psychology. This professional provides counseling for individuals with mental or emotional needs. A psychiatric clinical nurse specialist is a master's prepared nurse with advanced training in mental health nursing. This nurse may provide counseling or teaching for patients and families with mental health needs. Be sure that the mental health professional you work with has experience working with cancer patients. A mental health professional without experience in cancer care may not understand the physical and emotional issues and stressors with which you are faced. Your oncologist will be able to direct you to an appropriate mental health specialist. Remember, there is no shame in asking for this support!

## Legal Assessment

Your financial counselor should help by doing an assessment of your legal and financial status. Your team will ask about several legal documents that will help your doctors and family make decisions about your care. Specifically, your team will assess your insurance program, access to patient assistance programs as well as whether or not you have Advance Directives, Health Care Proxy, and a Durable Power of Attorney.

## Nutrition

Nutrition is a critical piece of your cancer journey. During treatment, you may have side effects that cause you to lose your appetite. A nutritionist or dietician experienced in cancer care can help you identify a diet that will taste good to you and provide the nutrition you need. There are foods that may interfere with your treatments or help boost your immune system; a qualified nutritionist will help you identify those foods. There are many cookbooks available with easy recipes for cancer patients.

> Be sure your healthcare team includes a nutritionist or dietician who can help develop a menu that is best for you while going through treatments. Ask your oncologist to help find the right nutritionist for you.

In addition to meals provided by your immediate support group, your nutritionist or dietician can help you find other sources for delivery of meals when you need them. Many communities have a Meals on Wheels program. To find out if there is a program in your area, visit their website at http://www.mealsonwheelsandmore.org/programs/. Check with your church or other local religious organizations that might have meal programs. Your social worker or nutritionist should be able to find contacts for you.

## Traveling

If you travel during cancer treatment, be sure to take a copy of your medical records and a list of all of your medications including brand and generic names, dose and frequency. Also, be sure you have contact information for your oncologist. If you have to get medical care while you are on the road, the information you can provide will be valuable to those caregivers who don't know you.

### Traveling with oxygen

Some airlines provide oxygen for therapeutic or medical purposes (often at an additional cost). There are also portable oxygen concentrators for flying, traveling or simply to do things outside the home setting. Check with your airlines to see if you can purchase inflight medical oxygen or bring your own. Either way, you will need a signed order from your physician. Make sure to plan ahead and check with each airlines for your options and arrangements.

Before you fly or visit a high altitude location, ask your doctor to perform a High Altitude Simulation Test (HAST) to determine if you will need oxygen when you are traveling.

Inogen is a provider of portable oxygen systems. Visit www.inogen.com for more information.

If traveling by bus or train, two weeks' notice is often needed for booking travel with a portable oxygen concentrator.

189

## Alternative / Complementary Therapies

If you do research about lung cancer, you will find a lot of information about alternative or complementary therapies. Complementary therapy is any treatment that is used <u>along with</u> standard treatment. These treatments may enhance the treatments prescribed by your oncologist. Alternative therapies are treatments that are used as a <u>substitute</u> for the standard treatment prescribed by your oncologist. These treatments are used instead of the standard treatments.

> Before using any complementary or alternative therapy,
> be sure to discuss the therapy with your oncologist and healthcare team.

According to the MD Anderson Cancer Center, these therapies may or may not be useful "...to promote wellness, manage symptoms associated with cancer and its treatment, or treat cancer. When properly combined with standard cancer treatments, some complementary therapies can enhance wellness and quality of life."[22] However, others may be harmful or actually interfere with your medical treatment. It is imperative to discuss any of these alternative treatments with your team as your complementary or alternative therapy may interfere with your standard cancer care.

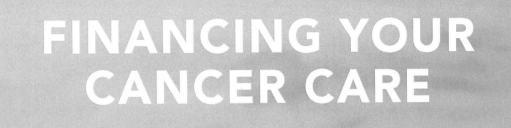

# FINANCING YOUR CANCER CARE

*The Foundation recommended
I go talk to another lung cancer
specialist up in Colorado—
Dr. Camidge. They opened the
doors to the right treatment,
but they also opened their doors
to their hearts. That's the best thing.*

*—Henry Randall "Hank" Baskett, Jr.,
survivor*

# FINANCING YOUR CANCER CARE

## Health and Disability Insurance

Your healthcare team should include a certified benefits counselor or a social worker who can help guide you through the process of applying for benefits should you become disabled by lung cancer. These professionals have been specifically trained to help you determine if you are eligible for financial help through your healthcare insurance or Social Security. You may also qualify for long or short-term Social Security disability benefits through the Department of Labor. The Medicare prescription Part D section may be available to you. If you are not eligible for Medicare, there are prescription assistance programs that might be helpful to you. Retirement or veterans benefits may help those who are eligible for them. State and community programs may exist including home-based programs.

When you are preparing to speak with a social worker or benefits counselor, be sure to have the following information:

- Recent statements from your insurance company
- Bank account information
- Medications that you are currently taking (for Medicare Rx or other prescription benefit programs)
- Veterans benefits and separation documents
- Retirement statements concerning benefits you are already receiving
- Social Security statements and card (if available)
- Disability benefits you are currently receiving

## Medicare

Medicare is the nationally sponsored program that guarantees that elderly and disabled Americans have access to health insurance and health care. You may qualify for Medicare benefits if you are aged 65 or older or if you have certain disabilities or end stage renal disease (ESRD). Your certified benefits coordinator or professional social worker can help you determine if you might be eligible for benefits. Your certified benefits coordinator or social work can also help you through the application process if you are eligible for benefits.

## Medicaid

Medicaid is the national and state sponsored program that guarantees that certain low-income families and people with certain disabilities have access to health care. As with Medicare, the process for qualifying and applying for Medicaid benefits as a lung cancer patient is extremely complicated. Your certified benefits coordinator or social work can also help you through the application process if you are eligible for benefits.

## The Consolidated Omnibus Budget Reconciliation Act (COBRA)

The Consolidated Omnibus Budget Reconciliation Act (COBRA) gives you the right to choose to continue your health benefits when you are no longer able to work. This coverage is the same as that provided by your group health plan and is available to you for limited periods. You may qualify under certain circumstances such as voluntary or involuntary job loss, reduction in the number of hours worked, and other life events. You may be required to pay the entire premium for coverage up to 102% of the cost to the plan.

COBRA outlines how you may elect to continue coverage. It also requires your employer to provide notice. For more information, go to the US Department of Labor website at http://www.dol.gov/dol/topic/health-plans/cobra.htm.

### Social Security Disability Insurance (SSDI)

The Social Security Administration (SSA) has a specific medical listing for cancer of the lung and a five-step evaluation process they will use to evaluate your claim. To find out if you are eligible for SSDI benefits visit the Social Security Disability program website at http://ssa.gov/disability/ or call 1-800-772-1213.

### High-risk medical insurance

Many states offer high-risk medical plans for lung cancer patients with pre-existing conditions. For a list of states offering these plans and how the new Patient Protection and Affordable Care Act affects you, visit the healthinsurance.org website at http://www.healthinsurance.org/risk_pools/.

### Special rates for the uninsured or for creating a payment plan

Many hospitals will work with you and your family to create a payment plan that suits your budget. To find out more, call your hospital's financial services office. You may also apply for a reduced rate for services such as diagnostic tests, treatments and other bills related to your lung cancer treatment.

### Patient Advocate Foundation (PAF)

PAF's Co-Pay Relief Program provides direct financial relief for insurance co-pays for drugs associated with the treatment of NSCLC. For more information visit their website at http://www.copays.org/resources/lung.php. On this site, you may also find helpful information for solving insurance and healthcare access problems.

> Note: If one of these organizations is not enrolling at the time you call or if you do not qualify for benefits, ask the organization you contact which organizations are enrolling new patients. Not all of these organizations are open to enroll lung cancer patients year-round.

## Patient Access Network (PAN)

The Patient Access Network provides direct financial relief for insurance co-pays for drugs associated with the treatment of NSCLC. You can sign up on their website: http://www.panfoundation.org/fundingapplication/welcome.php or call toll-free to 1-866-316-7263.

## Healthwell Foundation

The Healthwell Foundation may be able to help you cover coinsurance, copayments, healthcare premiums and other costs for some treatments. The Foundation supports a limited number of diseases at any one time and the list changes frequently. For more information on the diseases covered and the funding process visit their website at http://healthwellfoundation.org/or call 1-800-675-8416.

## Chronic Disease Fund

The Chronic Disease Fund assists eligible individuals with paying for drugs, co-pay assistance, and travel assistance. For more information visit their website at http://www.cdfund.org/Default.aspx or call 1-877-968-7233.

## Cancercare

Cancercare provides limited financial assistance, counseling with certified oncology social workers, support groups for patients and caregivers and community programs in Connecticut, New Jersey, and New York. If you live in one of those states, visit their website at http://www.cancercare.org/diagnosis/lung_cancer for more information.

> For assistance paying for drug treatments search online using the keywords "Prescription Assistance " and "[your state]".

## Pharmaceutical companies

Pharmaceutical companies may provide financial assistance to pay for drugs provided by the company if you meet certain financial requirements.

If you are having trouble paying for your treatment, check with your pharmaceutical company, local pharmacist or your oncologist for information on financial assistance programs. It is virtually always necessary to provide one's tax return for this process, so be sure to have a copy handy for the application.

*I see firsthand how Bonnie and this Foundation reach out and touch so many lives...lung cancer patients, survivors, and caretakers.*

*—Sally Samuels, survivor*

# END-OF-LIFE PLANNING

*It takes a family to support
lung cancer patients, and the
ALCF family is doing just that.*

*—Adeeti Ullal*

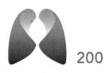

# END-OF-LIFE PLANNING

At some point in your cancer journey, you will be asked about the plans you have made for end-of-life care. You may have already created an end-of-life plan such as a will and Advance Directives. If not, we understand having these discussions now may be very difficult for you, your family and even for your healthcare team. These discussions may become even more difficult as you become more ill. Having these discussions and making these decisions early in your cancer journey can help you and your family feel less stress should your treatment plan change.

End-of-life plans include directions on how to manage pain, where you want treatment (e.g. hospice, home, hospital), legal documents such as Advance Directives and Health Care Proxy, as well as preplanning funeral services. Many of these end-of-life plans may be guided by your philosophical or religious beliefs and your spiritual advisor may be very helpful as you think about these issues. If your belief system requires or prohibits certain actions or treatments, your family and healthcare team must know about these limitations <u>before</u> the time when the decision must be made. If you have not made these plans before being diagnosed with lung cancer, it is important that you begin to think and talk about them and document your plans.

Although these discussions are difficult, your support system must understand what you want in order to provide the treatment you would choose for yourself. It is also important that these discussions continue throughout the course of your treatment; decisions you make at the time of diagnosis may change over time as your disease and treatments change. As your feelings about treatment change, you need to be sure your family and healthcare team know about these changes. By having your plans documented, you can relax knowing that your family will not have to make decisions when they may be upset...and that the decisions they make will be those you want.

You will also be able to focus all your attention on your treatment plan.

There are a series of legal documents to complete in order to capture your healthcare wishes. In order to complete the documents described below, you will want to talk to your family and healthcare team about what treatments and medications you want to receive – and at what point in your treatment you will not want to receive them. You may also want to speak with an attorney to help complete the documents.

## Healthcare Pre-Planning

It is important for everyone to plan for end-of-life – this is even more important when you are diagnosed with a serious illness such as cancer. End-of-life planning will allow you to concentrate on taking care of your health knowing that the rest of your team understands exactly what you want. End-of-life planning will also relieve the stress your family may feel because they will know exactly how you wish to be treated. As you review your end-of-life planning, the discussions may be uncomfortable at the beginning so it may be helpful to include your healthcare team, legal advisor, spiritual advisor, and your family.

A cancer diagnosis may carry with it a variety of legal issues, including insurance coverage, employment and taking time off work, access to health care and government benefits, and estate planning. These issues can be overwhelming to you. If you do not deal with these legal issues, you may find that even though you have made it through treatment, you have lost your job, home, or insurance.

## Online Resources

There are online resources that can provide great information as you begin planning. One very good resource is the Cancer Legal Resource Center (CLRC) that is sponsored

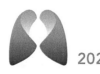

by the Loyola Law School of Los Angeles and the Disability Rights Legal Center. This center offers free information for you, your family, and your healthcare team. In addition to the online resources available at https://www.disabilityrightslegalcenter.org/about/CLRCEducationalMaterialsandSeminars.cfm, the center also offers support on a toll-free assistance line (1-866-THE-CLRC). When you call this number, you will be connected to an appropriate person (attorney, accountant, or insurance professional) to help you with your specific question.

The National Cancer Institute (NCI) at the National Institutes of Health is another good resource for end-of-life planning. This site will give you ideas about planning your care and managing symptoms at the end of life. For more information, visit the NCI website at http://www.cancer.gov/cancertopics/pdq/supportivecare/lasthours/patient.

## Important Documents

As you do pre-planning, you will want to prepare several documents. Although these documents do not guarantee your wishes will be followed, they will provide guidance for your family and healthcare team if you are unable to make decisions for yourself.

- An Advance Directive (AD) is a generic term that your healthcare team will use to describe a document in which you describe what medical treatment(s) you want to receive if you are unable to tell your oncologist what you want. For example, you may want to receive all treatments that are available to you – or you may not want any. The document known as a Living Will is a certain type of advance directive that may or may not be a legal document in your state. Each state has a specific format for the Living Will or Advance Directive. Your attorney will be able to help you determine the specific format that is legal in your state.

The AD document will also typically describe whether you wish to be resuscitated in the event your heart stops. A Do Not Resuscitate (DNR) order means that you do not want CPR if your heart stops. You can also revise this document at any time before, during or after treatment. Be sure your healthcare team has a copy of your current AD document. It is also critical that you discuss your wishes with your friends and family members. Let them know what your wishes are and how you want to be treated. It is extremely important to discuss your wishes with the person you name as your Health Care Proxy (see more information below).

There are online websites where you can quickly and inexpensively create a Living Will/Advance Directive that will be legal in your state. When you have completed the advance directive document, be sure to share copies with your family, healthcare team, hospital and health care proxy.

- The Aging with Dignity Five Wishes Online (www.agingwithdignity.org) allows you to complete the form online or print a blank copy to complete by hand.
- The Do Your Own Will site (www.doyourownwill.com/living-will/states.html) allows you to download the Living Will specific to your state for completion off line. This site is also a good resource for general information about wills and estate planning.
- Caring Connections is an organization that offers resources including a free Advance Directives document specific to your state (http://www.caringinfo.org/i4a/pages/index.cfm?pageid=3289).

- Your Health Care Proxy (HCP) document will identify the person you want to make *medical* decisions for you if you are unable to make your own. This person, or proxy, may also be known as your durable power of attorney for healthcare.

- The HCP is different from the Durable Power of Attorney. A Durable Power of Attorney (DPOA) names a person who has the power to make *legal* decisions for you. Your HCP and DPOA may be the same person, if you so choose.

In addition to the legal documents, be sure your health care proxy or family members or the person you most trust have access to information about all your will, living will/advance directives, credit cards, bank accounts, phone numbers, email accounts, investment accounts, and any other documents they may need in the event you cannot make decisions for yourself. We recommend you keep a file in a safe place that includes all these important documents.

Legacy planning is a wonderful way to leave a meaningful mark on your community and the world. As you go through this journey, you can discover many ways to make a difference in the world by leaving a gift to benefit those causes in which you believe. Giving a gift to organizations like ALCF can allow you and your family to leave a legacy that will touch others who are diagnosed with lung cancer in the future.

Our staff at ALCF would be honored

to discuss appropriate opportunities for legacy giving and recognition.

Please call 1-650-598-2857.

## Funeral or Memorial Service Pre-planning

While it is difficult to comprehend your own mortality as you are fighting to cure your lung cancer, some people find it helpful to themselves and their families to pre-plan a funeral or memorial services. Planning your service will help your family because you will make all of the decisions, sparing your loved ones these difficult decisions when you are gone.

The LIVESTRONG Foundation is a great resource for managing the pre-planning process. This organization provides many suggestions and resources that will walk you through pre-planning for your service. LIVESTRONG provides step-by-step instructions to begin the process and some things you should think about as you work through the plan. This site will give you information about funeral costs and different options for paying for the funeral. To access the information on this site, visit http://www.livestrong.org/Get-Help/Learn-About-Cancer/Cancer-Support-Topics/Practical-Effects-of-Cancer/Funeral-and-Memorial-Service-Preplanning.

## Palliative Care vs. Hospice

### Palliative Care

Palliative care teams are a relatively new formal concept in health care although the concept of providing comfort care is not new at all. In palliative care, <u>the goal of the team is to prevent and/or relieve pain and suffering.</u> This suffering might be physical, mental or emotional. <u>The desired outcome is always that your quality of life will be improved.</u>

Some people are confused about the differences between palliative care and hospice. Palliative care can be delivered at <u>any point</u> in your treatment including at the end of life; hospice care is typically given when the illness cannot be cured. Whereas hospice care is usually delivered in the home or a hospice facility, palliative care may be delivered in any environment.

### Hospice Care

While many people see hospice care as a last resort, we encourage you and your family to consider hospice as a caring support system. According to the Hospice

Foundation, "Hospice is the 'something more' that can be done for the patient and the family when the illness cannot be cured. It is a concept based on comfort-oriented care. Referral into hospice is a movement into another mode of therapy, which may be more appropriate for terminal care."[23] Visit the Hospice Foundation site at http://www.hospicefoundation.org/ to learn more about how to find hospice care in your area.

## Grief

Grief is a natural reaction to a diagnosis of lung cancer. <u>Grief is the emotional suffering you feel because your health and life have been changed.</u> The process of grieving is unique to you. Your grief will be influenced by your personality, individual coping style, diagnosis and overall physical health. Ignoring the emotional pain you feel will not make it go away. You might find that it is helpful to talk to a counselor or close friend about what you are feeling. Ask your physician to refer you to a social worker or counselor that specializes in cancer care.

The five stages of grief include:

- Denial – "The diagnosis is not correct" – This stage of grief is characterized by shock and disbelief.
- Anger – "What did I do to deserve this?" – This stage is characterized by feelings of resentment.
- Bargaining – Usually expressed as trying to make a deal with some higher power – "If you make this not happen, I will become a better person" – This stage is characterized by feelings of fear and guilt.
- Depression – "I am so sad/upset/down I cannot get up in the morning" – This stage of grief may be characterized by physical symptoms including fatigue, insomnia, nausea and vomiting.

- Acceptance – "I can deal with this no matter what happens" – This stage is characterized by feelings of relief and peace.

It is common to go back and forth between these stages. One day you may be angry and the next you may be depressed. Finding ways to cope with grief is important. First, find a strong support system that will allow you to share your feelings regardless of what they are. Second, take care of yourself. Eat right and stop and rest when you get tired.

Finally, do not be ashamed to get professional help if your grief becomes overwhelming. We are here to help. Do not hesitate to contact us at 1-650-598-2857.

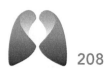

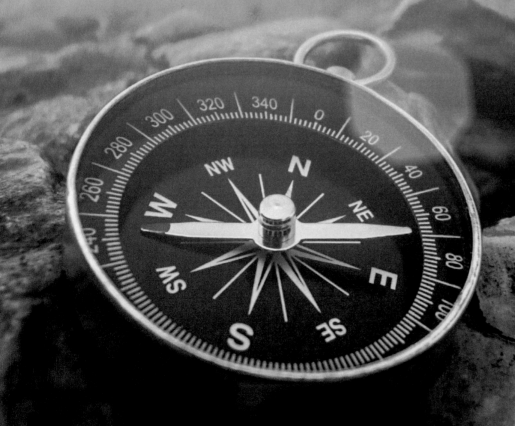

# OUR GENEROUS SUPPORTERS

*We're improving the standard of care by bringing new and improved treatment options to lung cancer patients. The future of cancer care lies in the concept of personalized medicine—a model that focuses on the individual, not just the disease.*

*—Bruce Gellman, Board Member*

# OUR GENEROUS SUPPORTERS

## Thank you, from the daughter of a patient

In 2003, my mom was diagnosed with lung cancer. Her life changed from one filled with business and family obligations to a life defined by doctor's visits, chemo and radiation therapy, and surgery. When my mother was diagnosed with lung cancer, my world changed as well. I was a wife, a mother, and an entrepreneur. Suddenly, I was the daughter of a cancer patient trying to support my mother on a daily basis while trying to find answers to complex healthcare issues. This guidebook is the culmination of years of conversations with patients, doctors, researchers…just about anyone with any information relating to lung cancer. I am grateful to our generous supporters without whom this guidebook would not exist. Thanks to their willingness to support ALCF, and the lung cancer community at large, we are getting closer to our goal of making lung cancer a survivable disease.

Throughout the guidebook we encourage you to call us with any questions. I want you to know that I understand the journey you are on and I am willing to help. Please feel free to call me with any questions.

Sincerely,

Danielle Hicks

Director of Patient Advocacy and Support & Daughter of a Lung Cancer Survivor

**As vital information becomes available, new print editions of this guidebook will be released with updated PDFs available on our website and through our mobile app.** *Check our website (www.lungcancerfoundation.org) or Amazon.com to make sure you have the most current edition.*

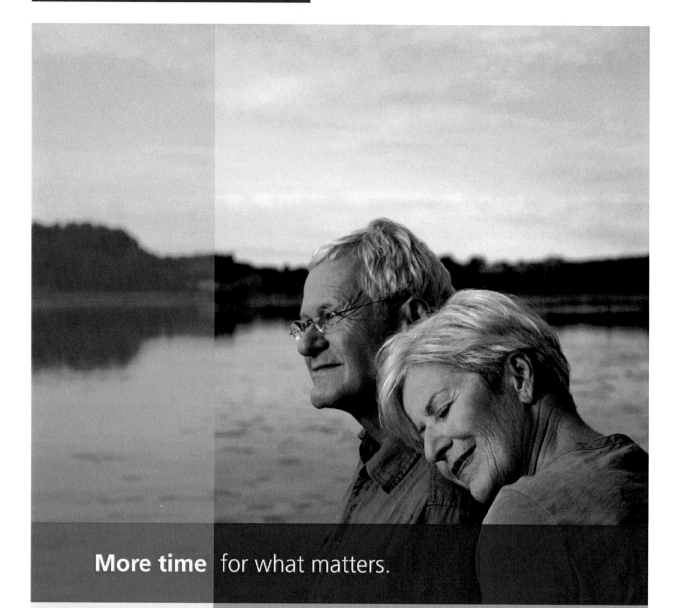

**More time** for what matters.

See Ben's story

When you have a spot, or nodule, on your lung, it's important to learn as much as possible about it. Fortunately, now physicians have a minimally invasive option for finding out what your nodule is and what, if anything, needs to be done about it.

See how the superDimension™ navigation system, nominated by the Galien Foundation as one of the Best Medical Technologies of the Year, made a difference in Ben Carlsen's life and how a quick diagnosis by his physician got him back to doing what he loves most.

superdimension.com/testimonials/ben-carlsen/

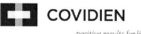 COVIDIEN

*positive results for life*

212

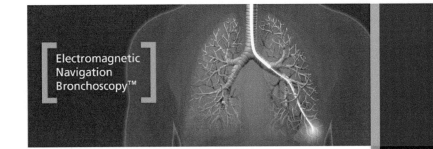

Electromagnetic
Navigation
Bronchoscopy™

## What is an ENB™ procedure?

ENB™ procedures provide a minimally invasive approach to accessing difficult-to-reach areas of the lung aiding in the diagnosis of lung disease.

## How does it work?

Using your CAT scan, the superDimension™ navigation system with LungGPS™ technology creates a roadmap of your lungs, like a GPS (Global Positioning System) does in a car. That roadmap guides your physician through the airways of your lungs to the nodule.

Your physician will insert a bronchoscope through your mouth or nose and into your lungs. With the bronchoscope in place, your physician is able to navigate through your natural airways to the lung nodule. Using tiny instruments, your physician will take a sample of the nodule for testing. In some cases, small markers may be placed near the lung nodule to help guide a physician delivering follow-up treatment or therapy.

## Who is a candidate for an ENB™ procedure?

An ENB™ procedure can be used with a broad range of patients, including those who suffer from poor lung function or have an increased risk of complications with invasive procedures. More than 70,000 patients have had the procedure, at over 650 leading medical facilities worldwide.

## What are the risks?

More invasive procedures come with a greater risk of complications. Pneumothorax (collapsed lung) is the most common risk. Rates can be as high as 40% for procedures such as needle biopsies.[1] Because ENB™ procedures are a minimally invasive option that use your natural airways, there is a lower risk of complications.

## Learn more about ENB™ procedures and whether they are right for you at: www.superdimension.com

1.    Cox J, et al. Transthoracic Needle Aspiration Biopsy: Variables That Affect Risk of Pneumothorax. Radiology. 1999; 212:165-168.

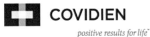

**COVIDIEN**
*positive results for life*

213

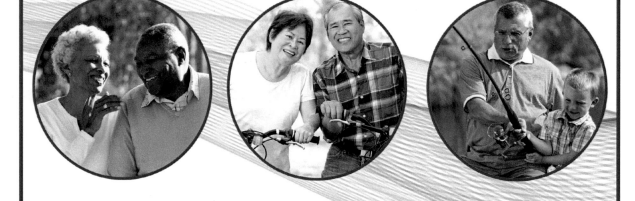
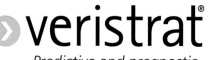

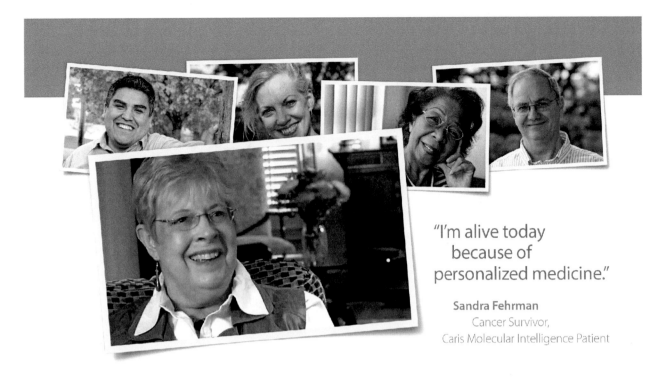
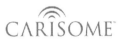
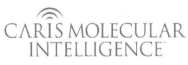

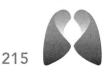

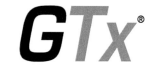

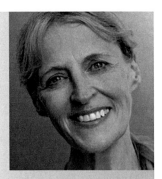
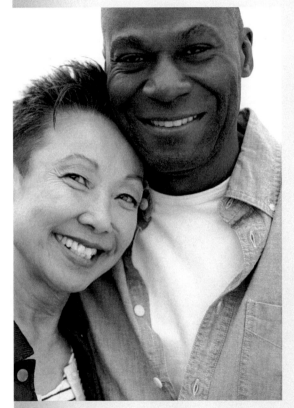
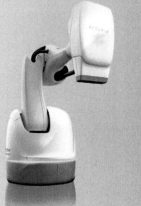
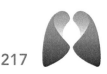

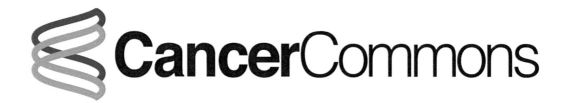

# CancerCommons

*"Cancer Commons puts the patient at the front end of a remarkable experiment...to work out personalized medical solutions."*

Dr. Donald Kennedy, President Emeritus of Stanford University
and Editor of *Science Magazine*, 2000 – 2008

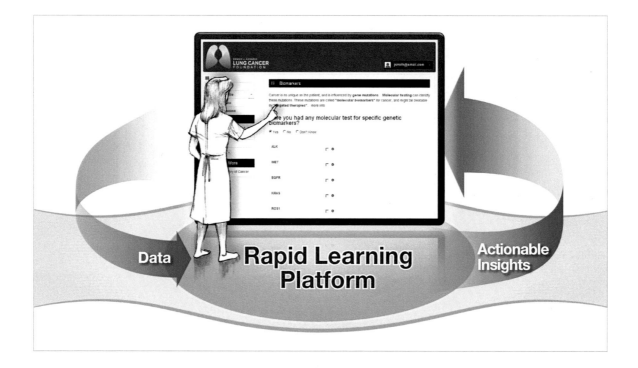

## Cancer Commons and the Lung Cancer Foundation jointly invite you to donate your data for research.

Researchers and physicians need patient data to test and refine their hypotheses about cancer biology and treatment in Rapid Learning Communities. The more you tell us about your condition, the better we can individualize the information and opportunities you receive. Please join us today.

## lungcancerfoundation.dyd.cancercommons.org

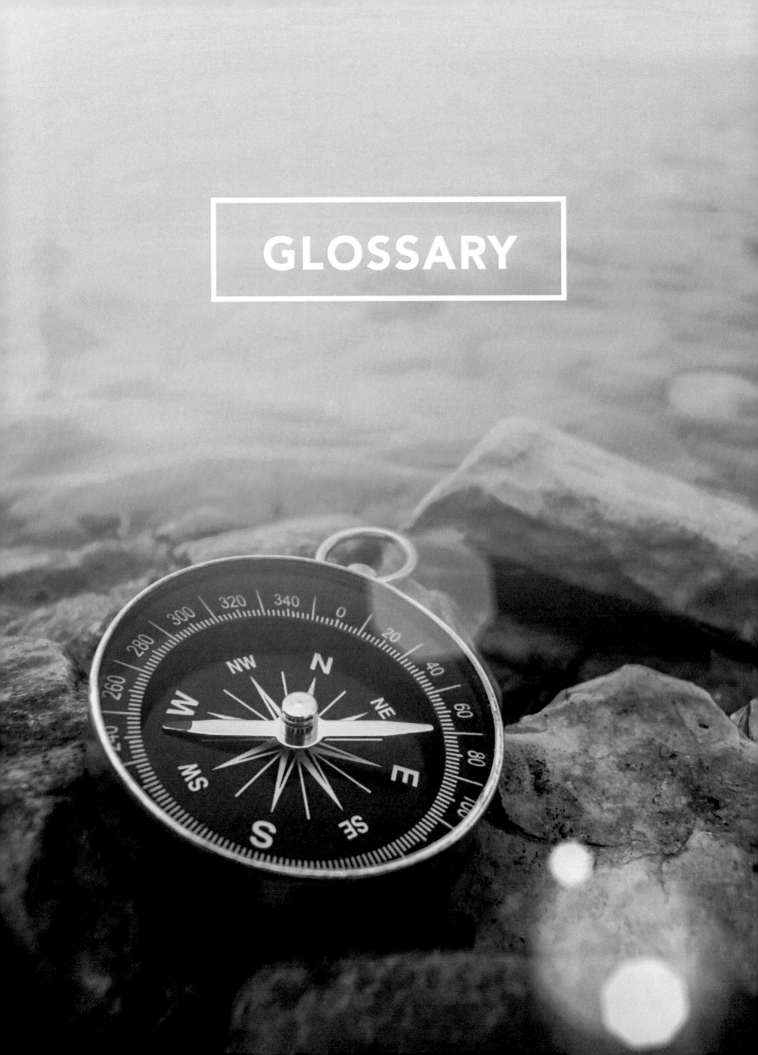

GLOSSARY

*I belong to this foundation and host a run every year in Gainesville, Florida, because I want to help all patients have a fighting chance to be warriors in this battle.*

*—Caren Gorenberg, survivor*

# GLOSSARY

**Adjuvant therapy:** any therapy that is started after surgery.

**Benign:** non cancerous

**Biomarkers:** biomarker or biological marker is a very distinctive substance that indicates a particular disease is present.

**Bronchi:** the trachea (windpipe) divides into two main bronchi which is a passage of airway that allows air into the lungs.

**Carcinogens:** substances that can cause cancer.

**Chemotherapy regimen:** a combination of chemotherapy drugs.

**DNA (deoxyribonucleic acid):** the molecule in every cell that controls how that cell grows and functions.

**Electromagnetic Navigation Bronchoscopy™ procedure:** also known as an ENB™ procedure, this is a minimally invasive approach to accessing difficult-to-reach areas of the lung using the superDimension™ navigation system to aid in the diagnosis of lung disease.

**ENB™ procedure:** see Electromagnetic Navigation Bronchoscopy™ procedure.

**Fiducial marker:** a small gold seed or platinum coil that is placed around a tumor to act as a radiologic landmark.

**Free radicals:** exposure to carcinogens may form molecules in the body called free radicals which damage cells and alter the DNA of the cell.

**Genetic fusion:** a gene that is formed when the genetic material from two previously separate genes are mixed.

**Genetic mutation:** a change in the structure of a gene.

**Hemoptysis:** coughing up of blood or of blood-stained sputum.

**Lymph nodes:** part of the lymph system that are responsible for filtering the wastes out of the liquid that passes through.

**Lymphatic system:** responsible for carrying nutrients to the body's cells and waste away from the cells.

**Malignant:** cancerous

**Mesothelium:** the lining that covers the body's internal organs and cavities.

**Metasteses, Metastasized:** cancer that moves from its site of origination to another part of the body.

**Molecular testing:** also called assays or profiles, can help your treatment team identify specific biomarkers that are in a tumor.

**Neoadjuvant therapy:** any therapy (chemotherapy or radiation) that is started before surgery.

**Next generation sequencing:** a technique or method of sequencing large amounts of DNA accurately in a short period of time.

**Pleura:** outer lining of the lungs.

**Pleurodesis:** a procedure that involves inserting a chest tube to insert chemicals to induce a scar, thus 'gluing' the lung to its lining.

**Primary lung cancer:** lung cancer that starts in the lung.

**Prophylactic cranial irradiation (PCI):** a kind of radiation treatment that may be used to kill cancer cells in the brain that may not be visible on x-rays or scans.

**Radioactive isotope:** an atom that emits radiation that can be seen by the radiological equipment.

**Secondary lung cancer:** cancer formed in another part of the body and travels to the lung.

**Thorascope:** a camera on the end of flexible tubing that allows your doctor to look into your chest.

**Trachea:** also known as the "windpipe," is a tube that connects the pharynx or larynx to the lungs, allowing the passage of air.

**Tumor:** a group of cells that stick together. Can be benign (non-cancerous) or malignant (cancerous).

GET INVOLVED

AND FIGHT LUNG CANCER AT

# NATIONWIDE EVENTS

# JOIN THE FIGHT

The fight against lung cancer requires vast resources, not the least of which is financial support. Whether through our national walk/run series, our annual gala and golf tournament, or the growing number of grassroots fundraisers, we depend on our supporters to help us continue our work.

So many of our patients, depending on where they are in the journey find peace, support and courage with others who are "standing up" for them in the battle against lung cancer. You are not alone. Browse through our events list to see if there's something to inspire you, your friends and family.

The money we raise goes to lung cancer research worldwide. It is our goal to turn lung cancer into a manageable diseaseby 2023.

# www.lungcancerfoundation.org/events

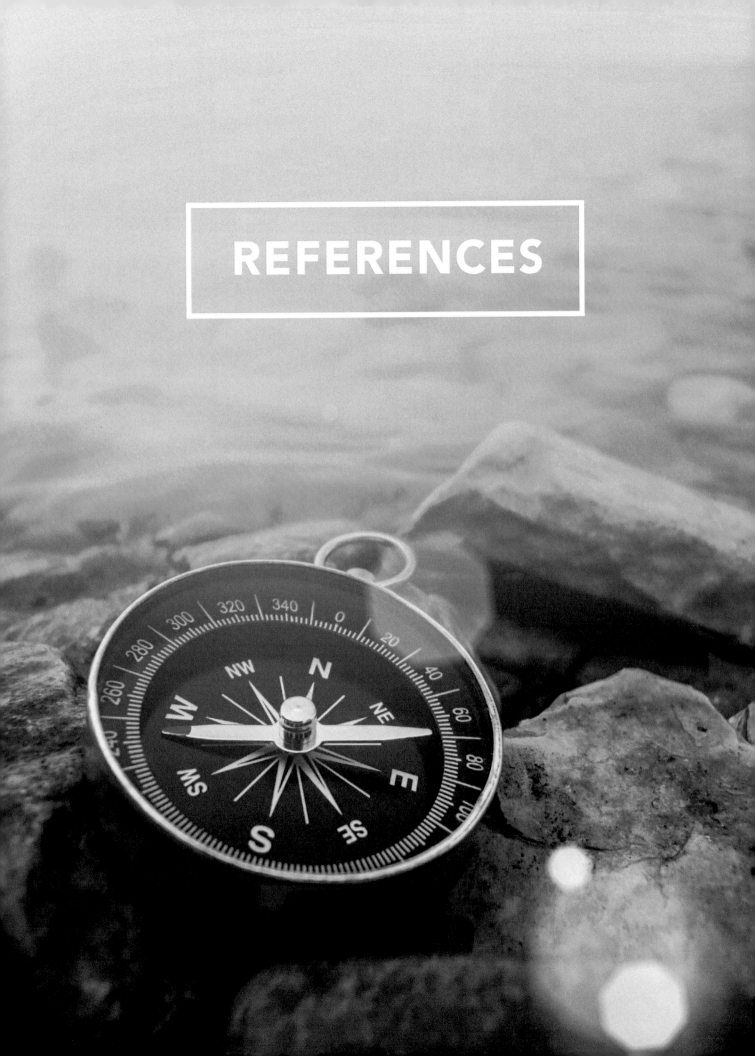

# REFERENCES

*I want to find a cure.*

*—Ellis Cox*

# REFERENCES

1. U.S. National Institutes of Health. (2012). National Cancer Institute: SEER Cancer Statistics Review, 1973-2009. Retrieved July 2012, from http://surveillance.cancer.gov/statistics/new_data.html.

2. American Cancer Society. (Oct 10, 2012). Lung Cancer (Non-Small Cell). Retrieved August, 2012, from http://www.cancer.org/acs/groups/cid/documents/webcontent/003115-pdf.pdf.

3. Read WL, Page NC, Tierney RM, Piccirillo JF, Govindan R (August 2004). The epidemiology of bronchioloalveolar carcinoma over the past two decades: analysis of the SEER database. Lung Cancer 45(2), 137–42. Retrieved August, 2012 from http://www.lungcancerjournal.info/article/S0169-5002%2804%2900054-6/abstract.

4. American Lung Association (n.d.). Understanding Mesothelioma. Retrieved June 2012 from http://www.lung.org/lung-disease/mesothelioma/understanding-mesothelioma.html

5. Mesothelioma Cancer Alliance. (November 21, 2012). Mesothelioma. Retrieved November 27, 2012, from http://www.mesothelioma.com.

6. American Cancer Society. (Aug 15, 2012). Lung Carcinoid Tumor. Retrieved November 2012, from http://www.cancer.org/acs/groups/cid/documents/webcontent/003117-pdf.pdf.

7. Sarcoma Foundation of American (n.d.). Patient Resources About Sarcoma. Retrieved June 2012, from http://www.curesarcoma.org/

8. American Society of Clinical Oncology. (2005-2012). Epidermal Growth Factor Receptor (*EGFR*) Testing for Advanced Non-Small Cell Lung Cancer. Retrieved June, 2012, from http://www.cancer.net/cancer-news-and-meetings/expert-perspective-cancer-news/epidermal-growth-factor-receptor-*EGFR*-testing-advanced-non-small-cell-lung-cancer.

9. Memorial Sloan-Kettering Cancer Center. (2012). Lung Cancer, Non-Small Cell: Personalized Medicine. Retrieved November 27, 2012, from http://www.mskcc.org/print/cancer-care/adult/lung-non-small-cell/personalized-medicine.

10. National Cancer Institute. (n.d.). About NCCP. Retrieved September 2012, from http://ncccp.cancer.gov/about/index.htm.

11. Goldstraw, P. (2009). International Association for the Study of Lung Cancer: Staging Manual in Thoracic Oncology. Denver, CO: Editorial Rx Press.

12. Nagata Y, Hiraoka M, Shibata T, Onishi H, Kokubo M, Karasawa K, et al. A Phase II Trial of Stereotactic Body Radiation Therapy for Operable T1N0M0 Non-small Cell Lung Cancer: Japan Clinical Oncology Group (JCOG0403) [Abstract]. Int J Radiat Oncol Biol Phys 2010;78: s27-8.

13. Timmerman R, Paulus R, Galvin J, Michalski J, Straube W, Bradley J, et al. Stereotactic body radiation therapy for inoperable early stage lung cancer. JAMA 2010;303:1070-6.

14. Chang, H.J. & etal. (2008). Risk factors of radiation pneumonitis in lung cancer. J Clin Oncol 26: 2008 (May 20 suppl; abstr 7573). Retrieved December 20, 2012, from http://www.asco.org/ASCOv2/Meetings/Abstracts?&vmview=abst_detail_view&confID=55&abstractID=34433.

15. Cancer Treatment Centers of America. (2012). Stage I Non-Small Cell Lung Cancer. Retrieved November 27, 2012 from http://www.cancercenter.com/lung-cancer/lung-cancer-staging/nsclc-stage-I.cfm.

16. Cancer Treatment Centers of America. (2012). Stage II Non-Small Cell Lung Cancer. Retrieved November 27, 2012 from http://www.cancercenter.com/lung-cancer/lung-cancer-staging/nsclc-stage-II.cfm.

17. Cancer Treatment Centers of America. (2012). Stage III Non-Small Cell Lung Cancer. Retrieved November 27, 2012 from http://www.cancercenter.com/lung-cancer/lung-cancer-staging/nsclc-stage-III.cfm.

18. Cancer Treatment Centers of America. (2012). Stage IV Non-Small Cell Lung Cancer. Retrieved November 27, 2012 from http://www.cancercenter.com/lung-cancer/lung-cancer-staging/nsclc-stage-IV.cfm.

19. Reveiz, L., et al. (2012 Jun). Chemotherapy for brain metastases from small cell lung cancer. Cochrane Database Syst Rev. 13;6: CD007464. Retrieved July 2012 from http://www.ncbi.nlm.nih.gov/pubmed/22696370.

20. Friedman MA, Cain DF. (1990). National Cancer Institute sponsored cooperative clinical trials. Cancer. 65(10 suppl):2376–2382.

21. ClinicalTrials.gov. (2012). ClincalTrials.gov A service of the U.S. National Institutes of Health. Retrieved November 27, 2012, from www.clinicaltrials.gov.

22. Complementary/Integrative Medicine Education Resources. (n.d.) The University of Texas MD Anderson Cancer Center. Retrieved August, 2012, from http://www.mdanderson.org/education-and-research/resources-for-professionals/clinical-tools-and-resources/cimer/index.html.

23. Hospice Foundation of America. (n.d.). Myths and Facts About Hospice. Retrieved online July, 2012, from http://www.hospicefoundation.org/hospicemyths.

- American Cancer Society. (n.d.). Understanding Chemotherapy: A Guide for Patients and Families. Retrieved July, 2012, from http://www.cancer.org/Treatment/TreatmentsandSideEffects/TreatmentTypes/Chemotherapy/UnderstandingChemotherapyAGuideforPatientsandFamilies/index.
- National Cancer Institute. (n.d.). Chemotherapy Side Effects Fact Sheets. Retrieved July, 2012, from http://www.cancer.gov/cancertopics/coping/chemo-side-effects.
- National Cancer Institute. (n.d.). Lung Cancer. Retrieved June, 2012, from http://www.cancer.gov/cancertopics/types/lung.
- National Institutes of Health. (11 Jan. 2011). NIH Clinical Research Trials And You. Retrieved June, 2012, from http://www.nih.gov/health/clinicaltrials/basics.htm.

1. Hagemann IS, Devarakonda S, Lockwood CM, Spencer DH, Guebert K, Bredemeyer AJ, et al. Clinical next-generation sequencing in patients with non-small cell lung cancer. Cancer. 2015;121:631–9.

2. Villaflor V, Won B, Nagy R, Banks K, Lanman RB, Talasaz A, et al. Biopsy-free circulating tumor DNA assay identifies actionable mutations in lung cancer. Oncotarget. 2016;7:66680–891.

3. Thompson JC, Yee SS, Troxel AB, Savitch SL, Fan R, Balli D, et al. Detection of therapeutically targetable driver and resistance mutations in lung cancer patients by next generation sequencing of cell-free circulating tumor DNA. Clin Cancer Res Off J Am Assoc Cancer Res. 2016;

4. Ali SM, Hensing T, Schrock AB, Allen J, Sanford E, Gowen K, et al. Comprehensive Genomic Profiling Identifies a Subset of Crizotinib-Responsive ALK-Rearranged Non-Small Cell Lung Cancer Not Detected by Fluorescence In Situ Hybridization. The Oncologist. 2016;21:762–70.

5. Cheng L, Alexander RE, Maclennan GT, Cummings OW, Montironi R, Lopez-Beltran A, et al. Molecular pathology of lung cancer: key to personalized medicine. Mod Pathol Off J U S Can Acad Pathol Inc. 2012;25:347–69.

6. Drilon A, Wang L, Arcila ME, Balasubramanian S, Greenbowe JR, Ross JS, et al. Broad, Hybrid Capture-Based Next-Generation Sequencing Identifies Actionable Genomic Alterations in Lung Adenocarcinomas Otherwise Negative for Such Alterations by Other Genomic Testing Approaches. Clin Cancer Res Off J Am Assoc Cancer Res. 2015;21:3631–9.

7. Lim SM, Kim EY, Kim HR, Ali SM, Greenbowe JR, Shim HS, et al. Genomic profiling of lung adenocarcinoma patients reveals therapeutic targets and confers clinical benefit when standard molecular testing is negative. Oncotarget. 2016;7:24172–8.

8.  Schrock AB, Frampton GM, Herndon D, Greenbowe JR, Wang K, Lipson D, et al. Comprehensive Genomic Profiling Identifies Frequent Drug-Sensitive *EGFR* Exon 19 Deletions in NSCLC not Identified by Prior Molecular Testing. Clin Cancer Res Off J Am Assoc Cancer Res. 2016;22:3281–5.

9.  Cancer Genome Atlas Research Network. Comprehensive molecular profiling of lung adenocarcinoma. Nature. 2014;511:543–50.

10. Campbell JD, Alexandrov A, Kim J, Wala J, Berger AH, Pedamallu CS, et al. Distinct patterns of somatic genome alterations in lung adenocarcinomas and squamous cell carcinomas. Nat Genet. 2016;48:607–16.

11. Ettinger DS, Wood DE, Akerley W, Bazhenova LA, Borghaei H, Camidge DR, et al. Non-Small Cell Lung Cancer, Version 6.2015. J Natl Compr Cancer Netw JNCCN. 2015;13:515–24.

12. Novello S, Barlesi F, Califano R, Cufer T, Ekman S, Levra MG, et al. metastatic non-small-cell lung cancer: ESMO Clinical Practice Guidelines for diagnosis, treatment and follow-up. Ann Oncol Off J Eur Soc Med Oncol. 2016;27:v1–27.

13. Arrieta O, Cardona AF, Martín C, Más-López L, Corrales-Rodríguez L, Bramuglia G, et al. Updated Frequency of *EGFR* and *KRAS* Mutations in NonSmall-Cell Lung Cancer in Latin America: The Latin-American Consortium for the Investigation of Lung Cancer (CLICaP). J Thorac Oncol Off Publ Int Assoc Study Lung Cancer. 2015;10:838–43.

14. Planchard D, Besse B, Groen HJM, Souquet P-J, Quoix E, Baik CS, et al. Dabrafenib plus trametinib in patients with previously treated *BRAF*(V600E)-mutant metastatic non-small cell lung cancer: an open-label, multicentre phase 2 trial. Lancet Oncol. 2016;

15. Sholl LM, Aisner DL, Varella-Garcia M, Berry LD, Dias-Santagata D, Wistuba II, et al. Multi-institutional Oncogenic Driver Mutation Analysis in Lung Adenocarcinoma: The Lung Cancer Mutation Consortium Experience. J Thorac Oncol Off Publ Int Assoc Study Lung Cancer. 2015;10:768–77.

16. Mazières J, Barlesi F, Filleron T, Besse B, Monnet I, Beau-Faller M, et al. Lung cancer patients with *HER2* mutations treated with chemotherapy and *HER2*-targeted drugs: results from the European EU*HER2* cohort. Ann Oncol Off J Eur Soc Med Oncol ESMO. 2016;27:281–6.

17. Li BT, Ross DS, Aisner DL, Chaft JE, Hsu M, Kako SL, et al. *HER2* Amplification and *HER2* Mutation Are Distinct Molecular Targets in Lung Cancers. J Thorac Oncol. 2016;11:414–9.

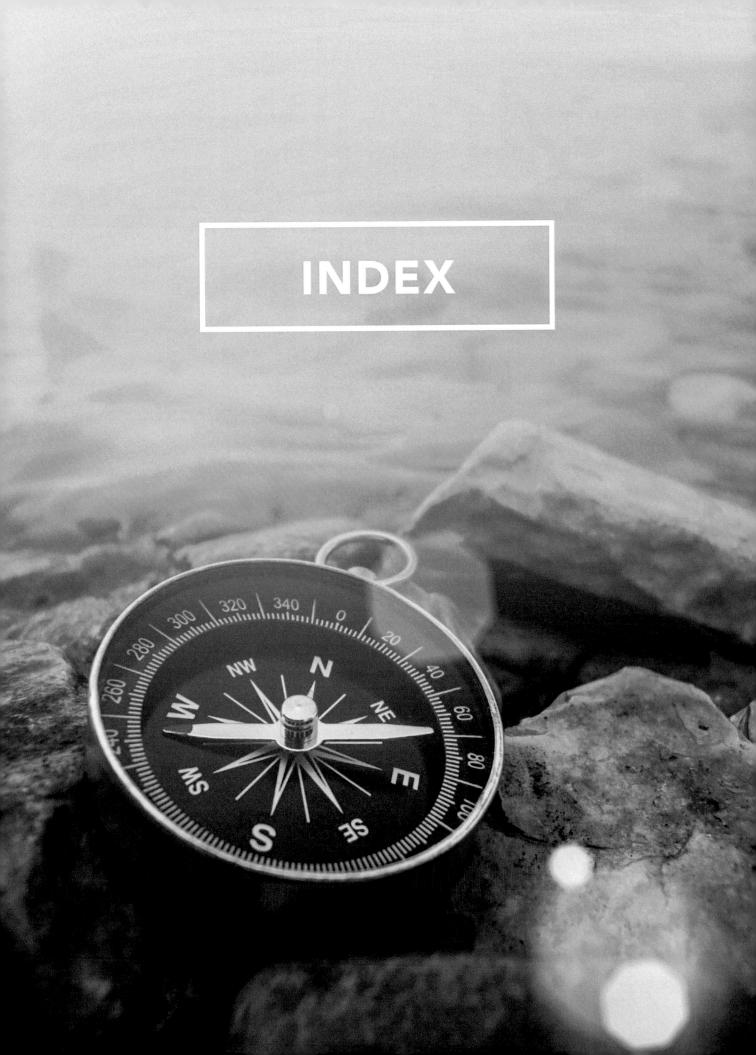

# INDEX

# INDEX

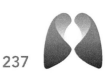

*The Foundation is a shining light to those diagnosed with lung cancer. They are knowledgable, helpful, dedicated, compassionate, energetic people—from the person who answers the phone (thanks Kim!) to every single person who is part of the Foundation! They go the extra mile and are making a difference for those diagnosed with lung cancer. As a lung cancer survivor, I am proud and so grateful to be on their team.*

—Jane Millman, Survivor

## SENIOR EXECUTIVES

Bonnie J. Addario
Chair & Lung Cancer Survivor

David LeDuc
Executive Director

Danielle Hicks
Associate Executive Director of
Patient Services & Programs

Andrea Parks
Associate Executive Director of
Partnerships & Development

Guneet Walia, PhD
Senior Director of
Research & Medical Affairs

## STAFF

Debi Beltramo
Director of Finance

Samantha Cummis
Director of Marketing
& Communications

Kendall Dempsey
Event & Database Administrator

Jennifer Hughes
Director of National Events

Leah Fine
Program Manager,
Centers of Excellence

Gina Tallerico
Event Coordinator

Emily Bennett Taylor
Spokesperson/Patient Advocate

Katie Wilcox
Manager of National Events

Michele Zeh
Manager of Patient Services
& Programs

Kim
Office Administrator

238

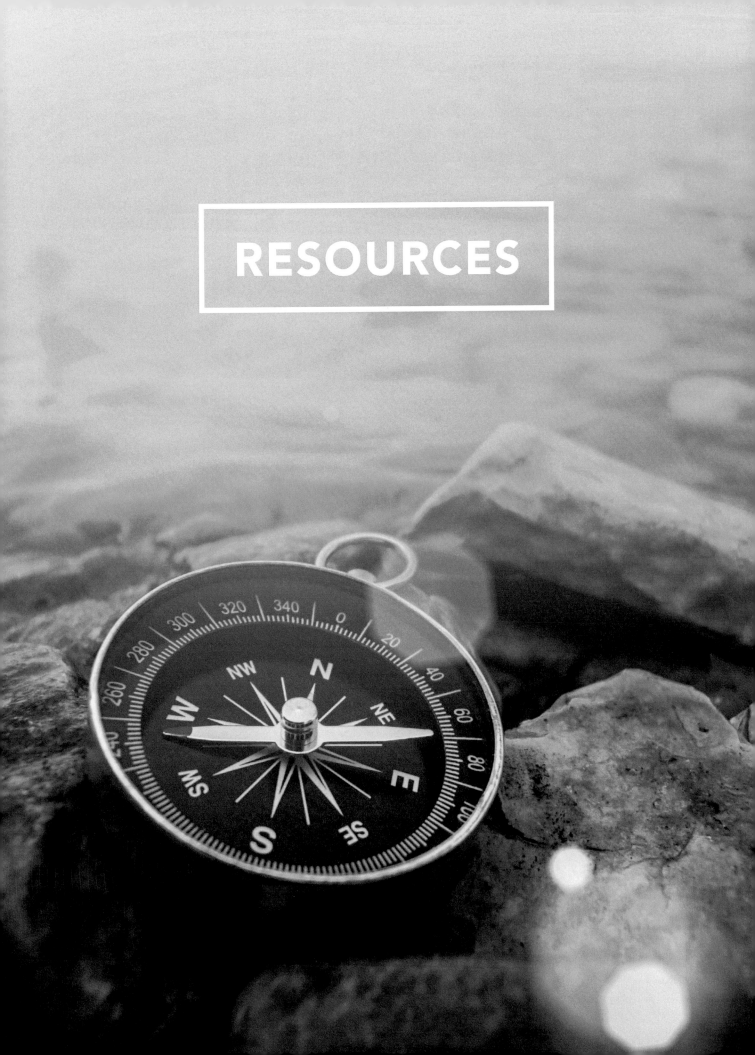

RESOURCES

Multiple resources exist across the nation to provide patients and families with medical help, social services, financial guidance, clinical trial information and advice about living with Lung Cancer (diet, exercise, etc). ALCF's list of Lung Cancer resources, both local and national, is a valuable for anyone looking for help in understanding and coping with this disease. Please visit their websites.

## LUNG CANCER RESOURCES
Bristol-Myers Squibb
Cancer Research Institute
Early Detection Lung Cancer Screening (I-ELCAP)
Mesothelioma Applied Research Foundation
National Cancer Institute (NCI)
National Cancer Institute: Map of Cancer Centers
National Comprehensive Cancer Network (NCCN) Treatment Guidelines
National Institute of Health (NIH)
OncLive
Radiological Society of North America

## RESEARCH EDUCATION ORGANIZATIONS
Caring Ambassadors: Lung Cancer
Free to Breathe
Global resource for Advancing Cancer Education (GRACE)
Lung Cancer Alliance
Lung Cancer Foundation of America (LCFA)
LungCAN
Lungevity
Uniting Against Lung Cancer (UALC)

## FINANCIAL ASSITANCE/INSURANCE
Bristol-Myers Squibb
Cancer Financial Assist Coalition (CFAC)
Cancer.net
CancerCare
Good Days
Lung Cancer and Social Security Disability Benefits
Patient Access Network Foundation
Patient Advocate Foundation (PAF)
Patient Advocate Foundation Co-Pay Relief
Pfizer: RxPathways

## DRUG ASSIST
Boehringer Ingelheim: Patient Assistance Program
Bristol-Myers Squibb
Celgene Patient Support
Genentech: Access Solutions
Lilly Oncology: PatientOne
Needy Meds
RxResource.org

## TRANSPORTATION AND TRAVEL
American Cancer Society: Road to Recovery
Angel Flight West
Bristol-Myers Squibb
Joe's House
National Patient Travel Center

## SUPPORT
Bay Area Jewish Healing
CarePages
Hospice Foundation of America
Imerman Angels
Inogen One Oxygen Concentrators
KARA
Legacy: Ex Plan
Livestrong Foundation
LVNG With Lung Cancer, a new site from AstraZeneca
MyLifeLine.org Cancer Foundation
Pathways
Stupid Cancer
The Empowered Patient Coalition
Tweet 2 Quit
UCSF Medical Center Bereavement Resources and Services

## CLINICAL TRIAL SUPPORT
ClinicalTrials.gov
EmergingMed

*I have been associated with the Foundation since the beginning. Here I am an 18-year survivor of Stage IV Lung Cancer who has really tried to understand the basics of lung cancer and its therapy options thoroughly. ALCMI and the projects we fund—any one of them—may lead to an innovative new protocol for early detection, a new therapy drug, or a new basic understanding of what lung cancer really is. This is an exciting time to be on the front lines of a science that can and will change very fast—and I, and we at the foundation will be there.*

*—Wells Whitney, survivor*

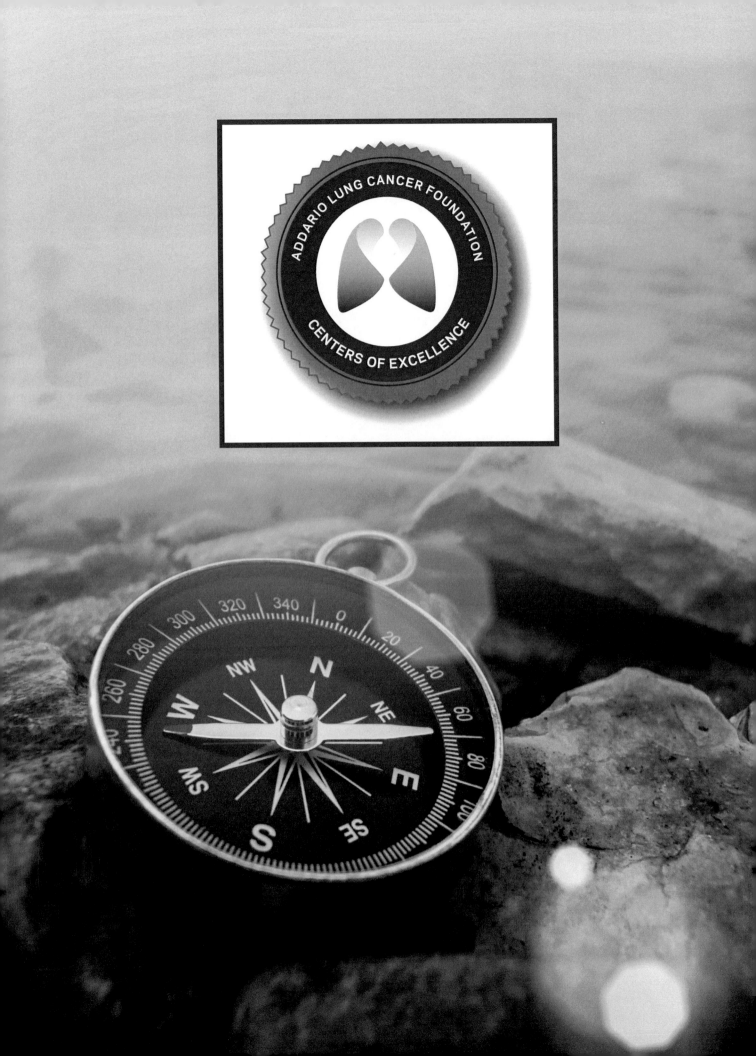

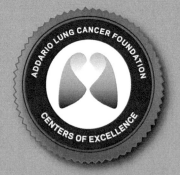

The Community Hospital Center of Excellence Program is rooted in the belief that the best way to treat Lung Cancer is through providing coordinated, multi-disciplinary care that integrates and considers the totality, the "big picture," presented by each individual patient.

# We consider the "big picture."

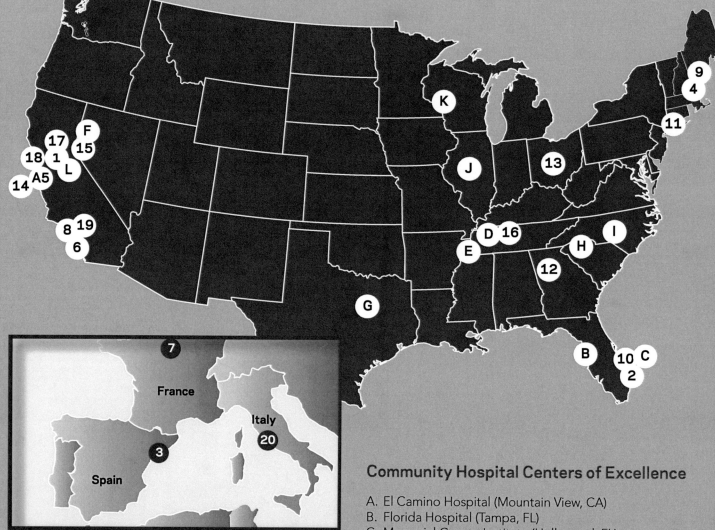

Brought to you by generous multi-sponsored support.

**Bristol-Myers Squibb**

**COVIDIEN**

## Community Hospital Centers of Excellence

A.  El Camino Hospital (Mountain View, CA)
B.  Florida Hospital (Tampa, FL)
C.  Memorial Cancer Institute (Hollywood, FL)
D.  St. Thomas Health West (Nashville, TN)
E.  Baptist Memorial Hospital (Memphis, TN)
F.G ene Upshaw Memorial Tahoe Forest Cancer Center (Lake Tahoe, NV)
G. Texas Oncology-Presbyterian Cancer Center (Dallas, TX)
H. Gibbs Cancer Center (Spartanburg, SC)
I.  First Health Moore Regional (Pinehurst, NC)
J.  OSF St. Francis (Peoria, IL)
K.  Gunderson Health (Lacrosse, WI)
L.  Dignity Health Cancer Institute – Mercy San Juan Medical Center (Carmichael, CA)

# ADDARIO LUNG CANCER FOUNDATION CENTERS OF EXCELLENCE

A critical part of this approach is the Community Hospital Center of Excellence Program, which is designed to accelerate lung cancer detection and patient treatment by utilizing the most advanced technology available to compassionate lung cancer specialists. Because 80% of patients receive treatment at their local Community Hospital, these are the centers where the greatest good can be done for the greatest number and we can improve the overall lung cancer patient survival rate.

Spearheaded by a pilot program led by renowned oncologist Dr. Shane Dormady at El Camino Hospital in Silicon Valley, ALCF is working with an elite team of specialists to create an unsurpassed paradigm for lung cancer treatment worldwide— a patient-centric, collaborative model to provide all patients, regardless of where they live, access to the newest and most effective diagnostic and therapeutic techniques.

This new "standard of care" established at Community Hospitals will be accompanied by a formal seal of excellence awarded by the ALCF and will ensure that no lung cancer patient is left behind.

## ALCMI Hospital Centers of Excellence

1. Alta Bates Summit Medical Center (Oakland, CA)—Andrew Greenberg, MD, PhD

2. Boca Raton Regional Hospital (Boca Raton, FL)—Edgardo Santos, MD

3. Catalan Institute of Oncology (Barcelona, Spain)—Rafael Rosell, MD, PhD

4. Dana-Farber Cancer Institute (Boston, MA)—Pasi Janne, MD, PhD

5. El Camino Hospital (Mountain View, CA)—Ganesh Krishna, MD

6. Hoag Hospital (Newport Beach, CA)— Doug Zusman, MD

7. Institute Gustave Roussy (Paris, France)—Jean-Charles Soria, MD, PhD

8. LA County Hospital (Los Angeles, CA)—Barbara Gitlitz, MD

9. Lahey Clinic Hospital (Burlington, MA)—Paul Hesketh, MD

10. Memorial Health System (Hollywood, FL)—Luis Raez, MD

11. New York University (New York, NY)—Harvey Pass, MD

12. Northside Hospital System (Atlanta, GA)—Howard Silverboard, MD

13. Ohio State University (Columbus, OH)—David Carbone, MD, PhD

14. Palo Alto Medical Foundation (Palo Alto, CA)—Ganesh Krishna, MD

15. Tahoe Forest Cancer Center (Truckee, CA)—Larry Heifetz, MD

16. Vanderbilt University Medical Center (Nashville, TN)—Leora Horn, MD

17. University of California at Davis (Sacramento, CA)—David Gandara, MD

18. University of California, San Francisco (San Francisco, CA)—David Jablons, MD

19. University of Southern California (Los Angeles, CA)— Ite Laird-Offringa, PhD & Barbara Gitlitz, MD

20. University of Torino (Torino, Italy)—Giorgio Scagliotti, MD, PhD

245

# NOTES

# NOTES

# NOTES

# NOTES

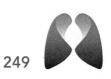